Achieving Excellence
in Medical Education

Richard B. Gunderman

Achieving Excellence in Medical Education

Second Edition

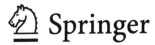 Springer

Author
Richard B. Gunderman, MD, PhD
Indiana University
Indianapolis, IN
USA

ISBN 978-0-85729-306-0 2nd edition   e-ISBN 978-0-85729-307-7 2nd edition
ISBN 978-1-84628-296-6 1st edition (HB)   ISBN 978-1-84628-813-5 1st edition (PB)
e-ISBN 978-1-84628-317-5 1st edition
DOI 10.1007/978-0-85729-307-7
Springer London Dordrecht Heidelberg New York

A catalogue record for this book is available from the British Library

Library of Congress Control Number: 2011925992

Cover design: eStudioCalamar Figueres/Berlin

Printed on acid-free paper

Springer is part of Springer Science+Business Media (www.springer.com)

Preface

A celebrated historian, a man who had won many awards for his writing, was invited to give an address at a great American university. In conjunction with his visit, the university's former president, a highly distinguished scholar and leader in his own right, invited him to lunch. As the two were dining, the former president asked the historian whether he had majored in history in college.

"No," the historian replied, "I was an English major. In fact, I did not take a single history course until my very last semester."

"That must have been quite a course," the former president replied.

The historian paused, looking at the trees outside the windows, "Actually, I do not remember much about it. I cannot even tell you the name of the instructor. He was not a faculty member, but a graduate student."

"So the course didn't make much of an impression on you?" prompted the former president.

"Actually, I was very inspired by something the instructor said on the first day of class," the historian replied. "He told us, 'We are going to be studying many different historical ages, events, and personages. As we do so, never forget that we are not just talking about names in books. We are talking about real, flesh-and-blood human beings, people as real as you and I.'"

The historian again looked out at the trees. "That really impressed me. I have never forgotten it. In everything I have written, I have always tried to capture the sense that we are dealing with real people, who got up every morning and laid their heads down every night. They were human beings just like us, who bore children, buried their parents, and who were in turn buried by their children. They gazed up at the very same sun, moon, and starry night sky that shine now above us."

"That's a beautiful story," the former president replied. "To which I would add one coda. The graduate student who taught that course?"

"Yes?" said the historian.

"You're looking at him."

Henry Adams, one of the great American intellectual historians, once wrote about teaching:

A teacher affects eternity; no one can tell where his influence stops.

Every educator was once a learner, and every learner becomes an educator. Whether we hold a faculty position or not, to practice medicine is to be a teacher. For one thing, the title by which our patients know us, doctor, comes from a Latin root that means teacher. Moreover, every interaction with a patient or fellow health professional is an opportunity to teach. We teach not only formally, with syllabi and curricula, but also informally, through the questions we ask and the examples we set.

Everyone knows that we learners model ourselves, unconsciously as well as consciously, after our teachers. We remember what we are assigned to study, we mimic the styles and phrasings of those who taught us, and when faced with difficult situations, we ask ourselves how our most esteemed teachers would respond.

Yet we sometimes forget the profound impact of learners on educators. There is a story about the behaviorist psychologist B.F. Skinner, whose students at Harvard decided to test out the theory of behaviorism on their instructor. During lecture, every time Skinner leaned to his right, the students would feign boredom, looking out the window or putting their heads on their desks. Every time Skinner leaned to his left, the students would show great interest, hanging on his every word. By the midpoint of the lecture, so the story goes, Skinner was leaning so far to his left that he fell from the podium.

Do students care about what instructors have to teach and how they teach it? Do they have learning objectives beyond the material that is going to be included on the next test? Do they realize that excellence in medicine has more to do with attitude, style, and philosophy than with facts and rules? Do they see that it is less about downloading, storing, and retrieving information than about imbibing and embodying character?

Do the members of the faculty come prepared to convey genuine curiosity, commitment, and excitement about their approach to health and disease? Do the members of the student body come prepared not only to memorize but to be challenged and inspired? What if faculty members never really invest themselves in the teaching, instead just reading their notes? What if students never really show up at all?

Education is like a dance, and it takes two to tango. Just because certain curricular material was presented in class does not mean that a faculty member truly fulfilled an educational mission. The mere fact that seats were warmed does not prove that learners really glimpsed what is most worth knowing.

Great education is like great jazz. To respond creatively in the moment requires attentiveness, playfulness, and generosity. Like great medicine, it cannot be preprogrammed. There is no checklist or set of algorithms or heuristics. Thank God it is not that easy! If it were, there would be no illumination and no joy in it.

Instead, there is only the promise. If we pour ourselves heart and soul into it, whether on the dance floor or the keyboard, at the bedside, or in the classroom, we may catch a glimpse of it. We are talking about something more than well-formulated learning objectives, sound pedagogical techniques, and high scores on high-stakes exams. We are talking about genius, something worth recalling and celebrating for a lifetime, perhaps longer. We are talking about a spark that we carry inside and, when conditions are favorable, summon forth to light anew, like the passing of a torch.

The educator? The learner? The learner? The educator? You're looking at him. Who can say where such influence starts or stops?

The purpose of the second edition of this book is to serve as the catalyst for reflection on excellence in medical education. What do we need to attend to make the most of the opportunities before us—as both educators and learners? What does real excellence in medical education look like, and what would be necessary to achieve it? What steps can we take to ensure that we pass on the torch of medicine burning a bit more brightly than when it was handed to us, and help each succeeding generation to do the same? It is my hope that each of these essays will serve as a starting point for medical educators and learners to engage in just this sort of conversation.

Acknowledgments

This book reflects the examples of many superb educators with whom I have had the privilege of learning. Each has illuminated the art of teaching in ways I am still struggling to articulate. They include Eric Dean, David Grene, James Gustafson, Leon Kass, Leszek Kolakowski, Paul Nagy, Robert Payton, William Placher, Mark Siegler, Norma Wagoner, and Karl Weintraub.

Thanks also to a number of people who have collaborated with me on projects on which this text draws, including Stan Alexander, Ken Buckwalter, Steve Chan, Mervyn Cohen, Janu Dalal, Josh Farber, Ron Fraley, Mark Frank, Darel Heitkamp, Adam Hubbard, Val Jackson, Ya-Ping Kang, Hal Kipfer, James Nyce, Aslam Siddiqui, Jennifer Steele, Jordan Swensson, Robert Tarver, Ken Williamson, and Steve Willing.

The Schools of Medicine and Liberal Arts at Indiana University have provided a first-rate environment for this inquiry. I would like to thank the deans of both schools, Craig Brater and Bill Blomquist, and the chairs of radiology and philosophy, Val Jackson and John Tilley, for their support. Thanks also to Lenny Berlin, Phil Cochran, Mervyn Cohen, Bruce Hillman, Steve Kanter, Bill Schneider, and James Thrall, and to Ruth Patterson for dedicated contributions to our shared educational work over many years.

Engaged learners are among the most effective educators, and I am immensely grateful to the thousands of students at University of Chicago and Indiana University who have taught me about teaching, as well as my friends around the world who have afforded me delightful opportunities to learn at their institutions. Finally, I extend heartfelt thanks to my most enduring teachers, James and Marilyn Gunderman, and deepest gratitude to my beloved wife, Laura, and our four wonderful learners, Rebecca, Peter, David, and John.

Contents

1 Education Matters   1

2 Theoretical Insights   17

3 Understanding Learners   41

4 Promoting Learners   59

5 Educational Excellence   75

6 Educational Technique   93

7 Obstacles to Excellence 105

8 Organizational Excellence 127

9 Center of Excellence 149

10 Educational Leadership 165

1

Education Matters

All who have reflected on the art of governing mankind have been convinced that
the fate of nations depends on education.

Aristotle, *Politics*

Defending Education

Academic medicine is like a tripod, standing on three legs. One leg is patient care,
one is research, and one is education. Over the course of the twentieth century, the
emphasis placed on each of these missions changed. In recent years, education has
become the short leg of the tripod. More and more attention and resources have
been devoted to patient care and research, and education has languished. This is a
dangerous situation, in part because it threatens to destabilize both medicine and
the healthcare system. If the profession of medicine and the healthcare of our
society are to flourish, we need well-educated physicians.

These changes are admirably documented by Kenneth Ludmerer in his 1999
book, *Time to Heal: American Medical Education from the Turn of the Century to
the Era of Managed Care*. He presents a scholarly examination of the major trends
in US medical education during the century, as well as a critique of the effects of
managed care on medical education. Ludmerer traces out the historical forces that
have placed medical education at risk, and provides insights into the remedies
that will be necessary to restore education to its proper stature in the culture of
our medical schools.

To appreciate what happened in the twentieth century, it is important to know
what medical education looked like in the nineteenth century. Ludmerer reminds
us that US medical education looked quite different then. Medical schools were
proprietary organizations, meaning that they operated for a profit. A typical course
of study consisted of two 14-week courses of lecturers, the second merely repris-
ing the first. To get into medical school, it was only necessary to be able to afford
the tuition. Many matriculating students were illiterate. Patient care was not part
of the curriculum. As a result, patients often suffered when graduates began "practicing" medicine.

Abraham Flexner's 1910 report, *Medical Education in the United States and
Canada*, spurred significant changes (Fig. 1.1). Flexner called for radical reforms,

R.B. Gunderman, *Achieving Excellence in Medical Education*,
DOI: 10.1007/978-0-85729-307-7_1, © Springer-Verlag London Limited 2011

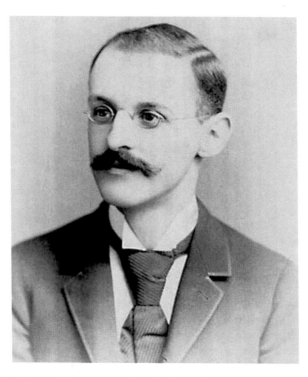

Fig. 1.1 Abraham Flexner (1866–1959). Though Flexner had not attended medical school or even earned a graduate degree, his 1910 report served as a catalyst for broad and rapid change in medical education, including the closing of many medical schools and the reorganization of both basic science and clinical teaching at those that survived. Through his work with the Rockefeller Foundation General Education Board, Flexner helped to raise and direct vast sums of money to institutions that followed his recommendations. In 1930, Flexner also founded one of the most significant scholarly communities in the US, the Institute for Advanced Study in Princeton, New Jersey, serving as its first director through 1939 (Courtesy of Wikimedia Commons)

including basing all medical education in universities, which he believed would provide the resources necessary to learn the scientific foundations of medical practice. Of greater concern to Flexner than the basic medical sciences, however, was clinical care. Many university-based medical schools were doing an adequate job of teaching sciences such as anatomy, physiology, and pathology. At virtually none, however, were medical students learning well how to care for patients. Flexner argued that students had to make the transition from a passive role listening to lectures to an active role actually helping to care for the sick.

The only way, Flexner argued, that students could learn how to care for patients was by caring for patients. They needed to do it themselves, not merely hear others talk about it or watch others do it. To do this, medical schools needed to be based in teaching hospitals. Flexner cited as his model the fledgling Johns Hopkins University School of Medicine, which had been founded several years after the

Johns Hopkins Hospital in Baltimore. Hopkins was the site where luminaries such as the three Williams, William Osler, William Halstead, and William Welch had introduced such contemporary staples of medical education as medical student clerkships and postgraduate training through internships and residencies. By allying medical schools and hospitals, Flexner argued, medical students would receive a robust education that truly prepared them to provide excellent care to the sick.

American medicine embraced Flexner's advice. The proprietary schools were rapidly replaced by 4-year, university-based medical schools that evenly divided the curriculum between basic medical sciences and clinical experiences.

This was the heyday of education in US medical schools. True to their status as schools, medical schools treated education as their principal mission, to which patient care and research were subordinated. Patient care and research were important, but education was the defining mission. Community hospitals could provide patient care, and biomedical research could be carried out in the basic science departments of universities and by research institutes and private industry, but only medical schools could produce physicians. The primacy of education among the missions of US medical schools lasted at least until World War II.

In the two decades that followed World War II, the focus of US medical schools shifted toward research. There was huge growth in the funding of research, and many faculty members began to think of themselves less as teachers of future physicians than as investigators expanding biomedical knowledge. Research became the most prestigious track on which a faculty member could be promoted and receive tenure. Medical schools and their deans began to keep score less by the quality of education they offered and more by the quality of their research and the size of their research budgets.

Beginning in 1965, another sea change began. As part of President Lyndon Johnson's Great Society initiatives, the legislation establishing Medicare and Medicaid was passed. Suddenly, the charity care that medical schools had traditionally provided, as a way to educate the medical students, became a viable source of revenue in its own right. Moreover, research was generating new and expensive healthcare technologies, such as the CT scanner. As the US healthcare budget mushroomed, medical schools began to shift their focus from research to patient care. In the early 1960s, Ludmerer notes, medical schools derived only about 6% of their income from the private practice of medicine. The social contract between medical schools and their communities meant that the medical schools would care for the poor in exchange for training the next generation of physicians. Poor patients would get free care, and medical students and residents would have "clinical material" to learn to practice medicine.

Beginning in the 1960s, this changed radically. Tens of millions of indigent patients were converted into paying patients, and healthcare as a business began to explode. Patient care, which formerly generated only 6% of the US medical school revenues, soon grew to over 50%, substantially exceeding both research and education. With the increase in revenues, the size of medical school faculties mushroomed as well. Between 1965 and 1990, the full-time faculty of US medical schools increased from about 17,000 to about 75,000. The typical medical school budget, which had been about $20 million, grew to over $200 million.

This great expansion in US medical schools was driven by something very much like the private practice of medicine. Traditionally, medical school faculty members saw only enough patients to permit high-quality teaching. Patient care was an academic endeavor, focused on educating medical students and residents. With time, however, medical school faculty members became less and less distinguishable from physicians in a multispecialty group practice. Medical school professors increasingly saw themselves as private practitioners of medicine, attempting to see more patients in order to generate more clinical revenue.

As the emphasis on clinical productivity increased, the time and energy available for education decreased. Medical students and residents tend to slow down clinical work, leading many faculty members to begin to practice in settings where education is de-emphasized, and in some cases excluding medical students and residents from the practice. What happened to research? In 1965 about 6% of US healthcare dollars went into research. Today, that number is closer to 3%.

As the scholarly faculty became a clinical faculty, another important change pushed healthcare and medical schools toward a managed care model. The people who pay for healthcare, including private insurers, government, and ultimately, employers and patients, became increasingly concerned about annual double-digit increases in the cost of healthcare. Between 1965 and 1995, healthcare costs rose from 3.5% of US gross domestic product, a level that was obtained for most of the century, to more than 14%. Alarmed by this trend, employers and patients began searching for ways to constrain and perhaps even reverse this trend. Managed care seemed a promising option.

In the old fee-for-service system of healthcare payment, hospitals and physicians were compensated in proportion to what they charged. Thus, the marginal revenue of providing an additional unit of service to a patient was positive. The more services a hospital or physician provided, the more revenue they generated. This system appeared to some analysts to provide an incentive toward overutilization, and thus to drive up healthcare costs.

What could be done? Some analysts suggested capitation as the solution. In a capitated payment system, providers are paid a fixed amount per covered patient, regardless of the amount of service they provided. It was like starting the day with a fixed amount of money to care for a fixed number of patients, and then taking money out of that pot as services were provided. This renders the marginal revenue of each additional service negative. Instead of rewarding providers for providing services, capitation in effect rewarded providers for reducing costs. For the first time since the introduction of Medicare and Medicaid, providers could actually lose money if they performed an additional procedure or kept the patient in the hospital an additional day.

Traditionally, payers had been willing to pay a premium for care delivered in teaching hospitals, in order to subsidize the education of future physicians. Everyone knew that teaching medical students and residents compromised efficiency somewhat, which increased the costs of care in teaching hospitals by about

30% compared to private hospitals. Every hour a medical school faculty member devotes to teaching is an hour taken away from patient care. Thus a medical school faculty member can see fewer patients in a day than a colleague in private practice. With the intense cost-cutting focus of managed care, however, payers became less willing to subsidize that inefficiency, and they began to cut back on the premium they paid teaching hospitals.

Suddenly, teaching hospitals could no longer compete effectively for their principal source of revenue, payments for clinical care. To reverse this trend, medical schools discovered that they had to increase the clinical productivity of their faculty members. Medical school faculty members had already begun to resemble private practitioners, but now they found themselves forced to compete directly with the most efficient private practitioners in their communities.

Ludmerer points out that the American Association of Medical Colleges defines the productivity of medical school faculty according to the income they generate. A busy cosmetic surgeon who never publishes a paper or teaches a medical student or resident appears to be many times as productive, and thus many times as valuable to the school, as a pediatrician or general internist who spends most of the day teaching.

This change in medical school revenues was paralleled by a change in the kind of care teaching hospitals delivered, with implications for the quality of education they offer. Ludmerer points out that in the 1960s, patients stayed in the hospital on average 10 days, and a busy night for a house officer was three or four admissions to the hospital. By the 1990s, patients stayed on average only 3 or 4 days, and a busy night meant admitting ten or more patients. Patients no longer came into the hospital to be diagnosed and then get worked up and treated. Instead, they were diagnosed as outpatients and then admitted for as short a time as possible to receive therapy. As soon as they could be discharged, they were sent home to recover.

The teaching hospital became more and more of a revolving door, and medical students and residents enjoyed less and less time to get to know their patients. The hospital increasingly resembled an assembly line, and the house officer became an admission and discharge machine. Ludmerer notes that the academic hospital whose hallmark had once been careful deliberation and attention to detail was replaced by a commercial enterprise whose principal mission was to get the patient out of the hospital as quickly as possible.

These changes took a toll on the resources necessary for medical education, including both money and time. In terms of money, medical schools were able, for a time, to cross-subsidize their educational missions from the clinical missions. The premiums for clinical care in teaching hospitals helped underwrite the costs of education. As those premiums disappeared, however, it became increasingly difficult to excite medical school administrators about teaching. Teaching medicine, which had once been the medical school's reason for being, became a financial liability.

Medical school faculty members who could once support their salaries through part-time clinical practice found themselves under increasing pressure to devote all their time to patient care. Ludmerer warns that medical education is returning to the proprietary model that Flexner decried at the beginning of the century. The fast pace of contemporary clinical work threatens to marginalize medical students and residents. If we are not careful, they will once again become largely passive observers of healthcare, rather than active participants in it.

The focus on clinical productivity tends to diminish both the frequency and intensity of educational interactions. The demands of clinical throughput sweep aside opportunities for hands-on experience, and student learning suffers. We can attempt to implement high-tech substitutes, but from Flexner's point of view, there is no substitute for learning by doing. Medicine cannot be learned at a distance. Not only is formal teaching under threat, but the opportunity for faculty members to serve as advisors, mentors, and role models is also suffering.

Ludmerer criticizes managed care as grounded in false assumptions about human biology. For one thing, the practice of medicine requires more than a science of health and disease. It also requires artfulness in negotiating with uncertainty. In particular cases, we cannot be certain that we have the right diagnosis or that we are prescribing the right therapy. If we attempt to provide medical care according to the same model we use for fast food, we will undermine the trust on which a sound patient–physician relationship needs to be based.

Without that trust, both patient care, and the education of future physicians who need to experience it firsthand, will suffer. If every patient arrived with a complete diagnosis and plan for therapy, then increasing throughput in our hospitals and clinics would not be a problem. But if that were the case, we would not need doctors, either. Because it is not the case, increases in throughput have been achieved at the price of diminished quality, which is harming both patients and students.

Is the practice of medicine a business? What if it is not? What if willing patients should never be subjected to tests and procedures, whether they can afford them or not, unless they are really indicated? Conversely, is it acceptable to withhold indicated medical care from patients merely because the payer would like to save some money? In each of these situations, we are purveying a defective model of medicine. If this is what the managed care prescription entails, then the therapy is worse than the disease of rising costs it is meant to treat.

Above all, we must ensure that our system of medical education, including our 130+ US medical schools, never ceases to serve the purpose for which it was created in the first place: to educate future physicians. Short-term cost savings are not worth it if they require us to jeopardize the long-term quality of our medical practitioners. Education is a core mission, perhaps the core mission, of academic medicine, on which the future of all of medicine depends.

Producing bad doctors lies in no one's long-term interest. Instead, we need to recognize the necessary ingredients of high-quality education and determine what sacrifices need to be made to provide them. We need to attract top-notch medical school faculty members, and to do so we need to make sure that we do not expect our faculty to work just as hard clinically for less money than their colleagues in private practice. We need to ensure that we provide them the opportunity to excel as academic physicians, including the academic missions of education and research.

Academic medicine needs to take the lead in developing quality and cost-effectiveness indicators, not only in patient care but in research and education. People recognize the harm that managed care has wrought on the academic missions, but we are not as equipped as we should be to assess those problems. High-quality assessments of educational outcomes are crucial. How do we know whether medical students and residents are being well prepared to excel as physicians, and can we track changes in the quality of that preparation over time? How can we demonstrate whether we are sacrificing quality to price? How do we know that our curricula are adding genuine value to healthcare? What really comes out of the time students and residents spend with faculty members, and how can we make that time even more beneficial?

How can we show the courage of our convictions, and stand up for the profession and the patients we serve when we see quality of care compromised? It is bad for medicine if physicians are seen to be caught up in internecine turf battles, protecting our own wallets. As long as we appear to be acting from self-interest, our efforts to establish performance criteria will be regarded with suspicion. Instead, we must strive genuinely to deserve the respect and trust that we once took for granted. We must rededicate ourselves to the core academic values that are the reason for the existence of our medical schools.

Ultimately, medical education can only thrive when the larger healthcare system reflects high-quality learning as a priority. We can indoctrinate students about the importance of patience and circumspection, but if they see us cutting corners and throwing caution to the wind, they will learn what we do, not what we say. We need to instill in our students and residents a clear vision of what excellence in medicine looks like, so they go into practice with their internal compasses pointing in the right direction.

But medical schools alone cannot reform the healthcare system. The best we can do is seek to regain our status as the conscience of medicine, and to reestablish our moral voice as society's healthcare prophets. If we are going to excel at these missions, we need to enter the public debate with unclouded vision and clear consciences. Nothing less will work if education is to regain its rightful place as the reason for being of our medical schools.

Educating Educators

We need to see in today's medical students and residents not only the future of medical practice, but the future of medical education. They are the medical educators of tomorrow. Yet faced with the daunting challenge of teaching medical students and residents everything they will need to know to be good physicians, we frequently forget to see them as educators. We treat them as passive recipients of education rather than future educators in their own right. This approach is grounded in part in a mistaken view that we must first become experts in a subject before we can begin teaching it. How could a medical student or resident who has been studying a subject for only a few years presume to teach it? How could they possibly compare to a faculty member who has been at it for decades?

Yet, teaching is not a prerogative that we acquire only at the end of a long course of training. Instead, teaching is an art in which we should begin to gain firsthand experience almost as soon as we embark on our education. We expect medical students and residents to begin taking histories, examining patients, and performing procedures before they have acquired full proficiency, because they cannot learn otherwise. Similarly, we need to expect them to start teaching even before they know everything, because otherwise they will not lay the groundwork they need to excel as educators.

We are kidding ourselves if we think that students and residents do not need to teach. For one thing, all of them interact from time to time with more junior colleagues. The freshmen learn from the sophomores, the sophomores from the juniors, and the juniors from the seniors. Likewise, the seniors learn from the interns, the interns from the residents, and the junior residents from the senior residents. Patient care is an inherently educational activity, because medical students and residents are continually called upon to explain things to patients, and to educate patients about their problems and their care. Why, then, do we not recognize such educational opportunities and do a better job of preparing learners to meet them? We spend countless hours teaching medical students about molecular biology, anatomy, physiology, pathology, how to take a history and perform a physical examination, how to perform procedures, how to find information, and so on, but little or no time helping them learn how to be more effective educators. By spending so little time on it, we send the implicit message that it is either not very important or there is very little we can do about it. Perhaps, we believe that we really cannot teach teaching, because we ourselves know so little about it.

If we understand better why it is important to prepare our learners to excel as educators, we will also illuminate what we need to do and how to go about doing it. When we gain a better grasp of the need to place greater emphasis on teaching, we also illuminate the format and content that such educational learning should take.

For one thing, education is an essential part of the covenant of medicine. To practice medicine is a privilege, both in the sense that society allows physicians to do things others cannot, such as prescribe medicines and perform surgeries, and also because those who enter it are entrusted with a rich legacy of knowledge and skills that were acquired through the blood, sweat, and tears of many great physicians and scientists over many centuries. When we enter the profession, we take an oath, often a modified version of the Hippocratic Oath (Fig. 1.2). That oath enumerates many responsibilities of a physician, both positive (pursue the good of the patient) and negative (do not betray the patient's confidence). But the responsibility that the Hippocratic Oath places first is the solemn responsibility to teach the art of medicine to those who follow us. The primacy of this obligation bespeaks the wisdom of the first Hippocratic aphorism, "The art is long, life short."

The art of medicine is far longer lived than any of us. It was here long before we came on the scene and it will persist long after we are gone. We are fortunate to be admitted to its fraternity, and we owe it to those who taught us, and those who taught them, to pass it along in as fine a form as we can to our students, and to prepare them to do so for theirs. The art of medicine is less like a stone tablet than a torch,

"I swear by Apollo, the healer, Asclepius, Hygieia, and Panacea, and I take to witness all the gods, all the goddesses, to keep according to my ability and my judgment, the following Oath and agreement:

To consider dear to me, as my parents, him who taught me this art; to live in common with him and, if necessary, to share my goods with him; To look upon his children as my own brothers, to teach them this art.

I will prescribe regimens for the good of my patients according to my ability and my judgment and never do harm to anyone.

I will not give a lethal drug to anyone if I am asked, nor will I advise such a plan; and similarly I will not give a woman a pessary to cause an abortion.

But I will preserve the purity of my life and my arts.

I will not cut for stone, even for patients in whom the disease is manifest; I will leave this operation to be performed by practitioners, specialists in this art.

In every house where I come I will enter only for the good of my patients, keeping myself far from all intentional ill-doing and all seduction and especially from the pleasures of love with women or with men, be they free or slaves.

All that may come to my knowledge in the exercise of my profession or in daily commerce with men, which ought not to be spread abroad, I will keep secret and will never reveal.

If I keep this oath faithfully, may I enjoy my life and practice my art, respected by all men and in all times; but if I swerve from it or violate it, may the reverse be my lot."

Fig. 1.2 The Hippocratic Oath. Often attributed to Hippocrates, the "father of medicine," the oath may have been drafted in Greece in the fifth century BC. The most venerable and best-known medical oath, sworn by many thousands of students each year as they enter or graduate from medical school, the Hippocratic Oath places education at the top of its precepts. What might be the rationale for this? Specifically, why might teaching and learning stand out as primary medical commitments? Educationally speaking, what sorts of lessons does the oath seek to convey?

and if one generation drops it or allows its light to be extinguished, it would take many generations to restore it. The better we prepare those to whom we pass the torch to pass it in their turn, the better for medicine and the patients it serves.

Education is also built into the very essence of what it means to be a doctor. The word doctor is derived from the Latin word for teacher. The verb is *docere*, which means to teach. Hence to be a doctor is to be a teacher. Before we can teach, we must learn, but it is in large part teaching that we should aim to learn, and to pass on to our learners. We cannot excel as physicians unless we teach well, and this is the spirit in which we should prepare our learners to be educators.

Great harm can be done by the misconception that we must be members of medical school faculties to be teachers. In fact, as we have seen, every physician is a teacher. Most of the teaching many physicians do takes place outside the classroom or teaching rounds, when we teach our patients and their families.

Our efficacy as physicians is not only defined by what we know. It is also defined by what we are able to get across to others, and in particular our patients.

We must also educate other health professionals, including nurses, social workers, respiratory and physical therapists, dieticians, and even chaplains. Do we do a good job helping them to understand our patients' situations, the nature of the assistance we are hoping they can provide, or where we worry we may have missed the mark? Being a good educator in this context means not only telling others what we do know, but also letting them in on what we don't know, and how they might help us. If our learners do not understand how to share knowledge in such contexts, they will be less effective physicians, and their patients will suffer.

In terms of professional flourishing, mere knowledge and skills are not enough. The physician who knows the most does not always make the greatest contributions, and the same can be said for the most skilled individual. Performing well also requires that we organize our thoughts effectively, focus on the most important points, and sustain the interest of our audience. These are traits of a good educator, and they are also traits of a good physician leader. Patients may not see our medical school grades or our scores on standardized tests. They may not know our final class rank when we graduated from medical school, or whether we were chosen to serve as chief resident. They do, however, notice how effectively we speak and write, and these are abilities that we dare not take for granted in our educational programs, lest they atrophy from lack of attention.

It is a mistake to suppose that educators are born and not made. To be sure, some people are more gifted than others, and others seem to face some constitutional hurdles in learning to teach effectively. Many anxious students and residents would prefer never to be called upon to speak in public. Of course, many might also prefer never to examine a patient or insert a central venous catheter, but we recognize that such skills are essential to medical practice.

Our educational programs should, as far as possible, prepare people to excel as physicians, disregarding what is easy for the sake of the necessary. Many learners report that it was the thing they felt most anxious about that turned out to be the most rewarding aspects of their educational experiences, in part because they frequently permit the most growth and development. Teaching involves a number of learnable skills, and if we make a sincere effort, it is one in which virtually everyone can improve. Not only does such effort make us better teachers, its benefits spill over into other aspects of our professional and personal lives.

Becoming a good teacher means becoming a better learner. The best educators know that teaching is one of their most important learning opportunities. There is an old Yiddish saying, "He who teaches learns twice." We never learn something so thoroughly as when we teach it. People who teach something for the first time report that they never understood the subject so well. It makes us dig deeper into the subject matter, and look at it from multiple perspectives. In explaining it to others, we see it better for ourselves. This helps us to set our cognitive bar higher when we study new subjects, because we have a better sense of what it really means to understand something well.

Teaching also helps us to understand better how people learn, including ourselves. Do I learn better by hearing or seeing? Which works better for me, attempting to memorize mnemonic devices or understanding the underlying pathophysiology? Do I learn best by trial and error or by imitating someone else's performance? Becoming a better teacher also helps learners become more effective consumers of teaching. They may be able to offer more constructive criticism of the educational programs they are part of, and play a greater role in improving them. Savvy learners are not threats to our programs, but key ingredients in the recipe for ongoing improvement.

The future of academic medicine, and thus of all future physicians, hinges in part on the educational abilities of the physicians we are training. Poor teachers mean poor education, which threatens the quality of research and clinical practice. We need to attract top-quality people into academic medicine, and provide them the knowledge and skills they need to succeed. Yet how can today's medical students and residents make an informed judgment about their prospects as academic physicians if they gain little or no experience with what academic physicians do? How will they know whether they like teaching, or are good at it, or would like to try to be academic physicians? By providing meaningful educational opportunities to our medical students and residents, and by helping them to succeed as new teachers, we can help to secure the future of academic medicine.

Some of the colleagues I respect most report that the most satisfying aspect of their careers has been the opportunity to help educate the next generation of physicians. It is one of the most profound and enduring sources of professional fulfillment. There is something intellectually and even spiritually rewarding about helping others to excel at the craft to which you have devoted your life. If we keep our medical students and residents so busy that they never have chances to experience teaching firsthand, we are doing not only them but also our profession a profound disservice.

What should we do? First, we should include curriculum on how to teach effectively in both medical school and residency. It is simply not the case that we know nothing about what separates effective educators from ineffective educators, and that what we know cannot be put to work to help people teach more effectively. Such information could be embedded in regular course work and conferences, or it could be the subject of retreats and other special events. Such learning opportunities need not always be presented by physicians, and in fact we in medicine have a lot to learn from other disciplines, such as psychology, about the enhancement of learning. What do good teachers do, and how can we use this knowledge to help learners enhance their own effectiveness as educators?

Second, we should provide formal opportunities to teach. Teaching should be a regular part of the educational programs of medical students and residents. We should also provide opportunities for trainees to receive constructive feedback on their performance, so they can improve as educators. Medical students and residents often do a very good job, perhaps in part because they are enthusiastic, the material is fresher to them, and their level of understanding is often closer than that of the faculty to the people they are teaching. Although residents and medical students should never be exploited, such programs provide the ancillary benefit of offloading some educational responsibility from faculty, who can devote their time to activities for which they are more uniquely qualified.

Third, we need to alter the criteria by which we evaluate medical students and residents to include their performance as educators. When we accredit medical schools and residency programs, we should look for evidence that they provide meaningful educational opportunities to their learners. Our specialty societies should make available grants for educational innovations that help learners become better educators. Awards from national associations might help recognize programs that do an especially good job in this regard. Research and innovation in education should receive more attention at many national professional meetings.

When we see that education is taken more seriously, we will be more inclined to invest our time and energy in it. This can spawn a culture change in which education is more highly esteemed across the board, raising its profile and enhancing its practice. When that happens, the entire profession and the patients it serves reap the benefits.

Developing Future Academicians

The future of medicine hinges to a large degree on the future of academic medicine, and it is crucial that we encourage some of the brightest and best among today's medical students to become tomorrow's academic physicians. Each generation of academic physicians educates its replacements in the medical profession. Both the majority of physicians who are in community practice and the minority who are in academic practice have a strong interest in securing medicine's future.

Yet we sometimes overlook the importance of academic medicine to the profession, our colleagues, and the patients we serve. The inducements to medical students and residents to enter community practice can be great. If we are to continue to attract capable medical students and residents to academic careers, we need to address explicitly the benefits of an academic career. What are the advantages and disadvantages of a career in the academy?

Community practice offers a number of enticements. One is compensation. In some specialties, community practitioners earn 50–100% more than their academic counterparts. Trainees feel this difference most acutely precisely when they are contemplating their choice of career. Most medical students graduate encumbered by considerable debt, and many students and residents are just beginning to face the financial realities of purchasing a home and starting a family. Hence, the extra initial income afforded by community practice is appealing.

The rate of increase in compensation is often greater in private practice, as well. Only a few years may be necessary to reach partnership in a community practice context, whereas academicians may wait 5–7 years to be promoted from assistant professor to associate professor, and another 5–7 years to move from associate professor to full professor. Benefit packages in community practice, including vacation, are often more generous. Community practice often enables physicians to utilize a broader range of their training. Healthcare tends to be less subspecialized in the community context. This enables physicians to see a broader range of patients. Academic practice, by contrast, is generally more subspecialized, and as a result, academic physicians frequently focus on a smaller range of clinical problems. Primary care specialties such as family medicine, internal medicine, and pediatrics are generally represented in greater proportion in the community context than the academic context.

This is reflected in the fact that patients are more commonly referred from community physicians to academic physicians than the reverse. As a result, academic physicians tend to see patients with more complex problems that are often more difficult to diagnose and treat effectively. Many college students choose careers in medicine because they want to care for the whole patient, and academic practice may present some greater challenges in this regard. When most people imagine a physician, they are likely to envision a community practitioner. How many premedical students are drawn to careers in medicine because they want to be medical researchers or medical educators? They are more likely to have in mind the image of community physicians who devote the bulk of their time and energy to caring for patients. If they have no firsthand experience with teaching or research, and if their medical school provides no experience with these pursuits, it is no wonder that many of them do not see themselves as educators or researchers.

They may find acquiring the knowledge and skills necessary to care well for patients a daunting prospect in itself, and have no desire to take on the additional responsibilities of an academic physician. Likewise, teaching and conducting research may seem like distractions from their primary calling as physicians that might interfere with their ability to be good doctors. The community physician can succeed by being a good physician, whereas the academic physician frequently needs to thrive in other spheres as well, and many students are not enticed by the prospect of assuming those additional responsibilities. Moreover, it is of course possible for community physicians to engage in teaching and research, but without the more stringent promotion and tenure requirements of an academic career.

Another frequent advantage of community practice is autonomy. Although solo practice is a less common option than in the past, many primary care physicians still operate largely independent practices. Even those in group practices usually enjoy a large degree of influence over how their practice operates. They are often part owners of their practice, and play an active role in determining who they work with, setting the group's priorities, and measuring its success. By contrast, most full-time academicians function within large bureaucracies, where each faculty member enjoys relatively less influence in deciding what the medical school does.

The opportunity to play an active role in shaping the work environments of one's self and one's colleagues may be an important factor in career choice for many medical students and residents, and they may reasonably conclude that community practice offers more opportunities in this regard. Of course, not all community physicians are part of physician-owned groups, and all community practice groups do not operate according to such a participative model. Moreover, some medical schools adopt a more democratic model of governance that invites a greater degree of participation and leadership by individual faculty members. In general, however, community practitioners tend to enjoy a greater degree of professional autonomy.

The economics of medicine have tended to blur the lines between community practice and academic practice. In an effort to sustain and augment their revenues, many academic health centers have developed clinical tracks for their faculty, which resemble community practice. Faculty members are hired, retained, and promoted to an increasing degree based on their clinical performance, with research and even teaching playing little or no role.

As the fiscal health of the medical school depends more and more on its faculty's clinical productivity, it has incentivized its faculty to focus more and more on clinical work. For community practitioners, this would mean simply increasing the efficiency of what they are already doing. For academic physicians, it means reallocating time and effort away from traditional academic pursuits. This, in turn, may render it more difficult to succeed as an academic physician. If academic practice is becoming more like community practice, and if academic physicians enjoy less autonomy and lower levels of compensation, many trainees might find academic practice less attractive.

What are the advantages of academic practice? In many cases, academic environments are especially conducive to state-of-the-art clinical practice. As centers for research and innovation, academic health centers foster an appetite for new ways of doing things. Bench research, translational research, and clinical trials are more likely to be conducted in academic centers. Many faculty members see themselves primarily as researchers, and their careers depend on their ability to discover and innovate. The bulk of extramural funding at many academic centers is targeted at research. Academic centers are more likely to offer regular research presentations and to conduct journal clubs. As a result, academic centers focus relatively less on applying to patient care the information already contained in the textbooks, and relatively more on writing the journal articles and textbooks of tomorrow. Medical students and residents who find research and innovation an attractive prospect may find academic health centers a more hospitable environment.

This attitude also manifests itself in everyday clinical practice, where academicians are often somewhat more self-critical and may seek to ground their practice to a greater degree in scientific evidence. They often manifest a greater tolerance and appetite for asking questions. Many of the most widely recognized experts and opinion leaders in the different medical fields are academic physicians, and it is often to academic centers that physicians refer their most difficult cases. Many new diagnostic tests, medical therapies, and devices were developed by academic physicians, who were privileged to experience the deep satisfaction that comes from seeing your work embodied in the daily practice of others.

Education is another distinctive pursuit of academic physicians. Every physician who cares for patients is an educator, but working in an environment heavily populated by medical students, residents, and fellows places a special premium on playing the educational role for academic physicians. Teaching is an essential aspect of being a physician. For many physicians, teaching turns out to be one of the most rewarding aspects of their medical career, the one they look back on with the most pride.

It is an awesome responsibility to help educate the next generation of physicians to whom the torch of medicine will be passed, and doing so well takes a great deal of effort. Yet when it goes well, it is also immensely satisfying. It recognizes and strengthens a powerful human link between generations that binds us to the generations of physicians who preceded us, and will live on in the generations yet to come. If we do not do a good job of educating the physicians of tomorrow, who will?

Educational excellence is important not merely because it opens up doors to promotion and tenure. It is important because those who can teach a subject well generally enjoy a deeper understanding of it than those who cannot. In the course of teaching, we are invited to reexamine what we think we know, to discover things that we thought we knew but do not, and to make new connections between the things we know. Learners ask good questions, and putting what we know in a way that a novice could understand helps distill and clarify what we might otherwise merely take for granted. The opportunity to teach is a great privilege in part because teaching is a portal to greater understanding. The educator needs to stay on top of new developments in the field, and to integrate them into current models of practice.

From a service perspective, academic practice offers important opportunities. In many medical fields, academic physicians tend to be overrepresented in the governance of professional organizations. Because the next generation of specialists in any field is trained largely in medical schools, faculty members enjoy special opportunities to influence their field's future. Academic physicians tend to see themselves as setting the intellectual agenda for their field, and as a result, are more likely to see service in such organizations as part of their professional mission. Academic physicians can influence not only medical schools but the larger universities of which they are a part, and thus make contributions to higher education as a whole.

If academic medicine is going to thrive in the future, it is vital that medical schools and residency programs provide their trainees with meaningful opportunities to experience firsthand what it is like to be an academic physician. If learners do not experience academic medicine in this way, they will be unable to make fully informed choices about what kind of medical practice they wish to pursue. The special challenges and rewards of academic medicine may be largely unknown to them, and they may fail to consider a career path to which, in some cases, they may be very well suited. What is it like to augment the body of knowledge relied upon by physicians around the world? What is it like to see the curiosity of a medical student or resident ignited by a question you have posed? What is it like to help make a significant improvement in the way future physicians are trained? With more and more time and energy devoted to clinical practice, faculty time to support such opportunities is becoming scarcer.

We need to evaluate our level of commitment to the academic enterprise, and be prepared to fight for that in which we believe. Are medicine's academic missions sufficiently important to us that we are prepared to develop and preserve extra revenue sources for academic medical centers? In the past, healthcare payers recognized that it costs more to deliver care in academic centers, in part because patients tend to be sicker to be able to contribute less financially to their own care, and because teaching slows down the process of clinical care.

How important is it to us to continue to advance medical knowledge at a rapid pace and to provide a superb educational experience for the health professionals of tomorrow? Are we prepared to provide the resources for first-rate education and research? It is not enough to attract bright people into academic careers. We must provide them the time, tools, and intellectual environments they need to thrive, year after year. This is a concern not only for academic physicians, but for physicians in community practice as well, because the long-term future of medicine as a whole hinges on the work done in academic health centers. Investing in academic medicine is like planting trees—it takes years or even decades before we see the fruits of our labors.

To foster the best academic physicians, we should encourage our learners to reflect from time to time on the kinds of physicians they want to become. How important is it to them to be actively engaged in the pursuit of knowledge? Would they find teaching the next generation of physicians a rewarding pursuit? Do they wish to make special leadership contributions to their field? How important is it to them to be a good doctor for their patients, and what proportion of their time do they wish to devote to patient care? Where would they rank income as a priority, and how much money do they need to be happy? We should not pretend that academic practice is right for everyone, but for those with special interests and aptitudes in the distinctively academic pursuits, it offers a marvelous opportunity for deep professional engagement and fulfillment.

2

Theoretical Insights

> We are only just realizing that the art and science of education require a genius and a study of their own; and that this genius and this science are more than a bare knowledge of some branch of science or literature.
>
> Alfred North Whitehead, *The Aims of Education*

Learning Theory in Medical Education

If medical educators are to perform at our best, it is vital that we understand how people learn. Learning, not teaching, is the ultimate outcome of medical education, and we are unlikely to foster it effectively if we do not understand what it is and how it takes place. Yet most medical educators have little or no background in formal educational theory. If we are good teachers, it is frequently because we were blessed with good educational instincts, or because we had the good fortune to study with and emulate other good teachers. We need not leave our capabilities as teachers entirely to chance, however. Those of us who are not particularly accomplished educators can learn a great deal from the educational literature, and even those who are already very good can hone our skills even further. Happily, thoughtful people have been studying learning for many years, and important insights are readily available, if only we are prepared to look beyond the boundaries of our own field.

This section reviews four important learning theories that powerfully influenced educational practice during the twentieth century. They are not the only learning theories that were developed during this period of time, nor were they necessarily the most important. They do, however, provide a broad overview of the spectrum of theoretical approaches to learning. The very fact that there are four theories indicates that no single one has achieved universal dominance.

Unlike Newton's theory of gravitation, which largely put to rest attempts to develop alternative explanations for the attraction between objects, educational theorists have not achieved a single consensus. Each of the theories has its own strengths and weaknesses, and no one answers all questions. The purpose in presenting four different theories is not to suggest that we must choose one and completely eliminate the other three. Instead, each illuminates certain aspects of learning, and may provide valuable insights in certain situations. The goal in

R.B. Gunderman, *Achieving Excellence in Medical Education*,
DOI: 10.1007/978-0-85729-307-7_2, © Springer-Verlag London Limited 2011

reviewing these theories is to provoke our own reflective educational practice, and to inspire new approaches that improve our educational efficiency and effectiveness. Efficiency refers to the resources expended to achieve a particular goal. They may include time, effort, personnel (educator full-time equivalents [FTEs]), money, and so on. If we can achieve the same educational results with a lower expenditure of resources, then we have improved our educational efficiency.

For example, it might turn out that medical students can learn certain aspects of human anatomy using an interactive computer-based anatomy tutorial as well as when working one-on-one with an anatomy tutor. If that is the case, and if the computer-based tutorial requires substantially fewer person-hours of instructor time, then it offers greater educational efficiency. Effectiveness, by contrast, refers to the quality of the educational result; that is, what the learners actually take away from learning activities. If we better understand how we learn, we should be able to enhance the quality of education we offer. To a substantial degree, our implicit, perhaps even inchoate, theories of learning shape our educational practice. What are we trying to teach? How are we trying to teach it? How do we determine whether learners have learned it? The answers to these questions reflect our understanding of the nature of learning itself. What we are trying to teach is often referred to as curriculum. At first, curriculum seems quite straightforward, but it can be divided into at least two components: the formal curriculum and the informal curriculum.

The formal curriculum consists of the reading assignments, lectures, and other learning activities formally assigned to learners. In addition to the formal curriculum, there is also an informal curriculum, which consists of what learners learn that educators do not explicitly tell them to learn. For example, medical students and residents learn by observing how to interact with other health professionals, how to handle failure, and how to balance their professional and personal lives. Our sense of the boundaries between the formal and informal curriculum, as well as the content of each, is powerfully shaped by our theoretical perspective on learning.

How we teach is often referred to as instruction. What is our instructional approach? Do we think of instruction as consisting primarily of what we ask learners to read? Do we expect learners to learn primarily by doing? To what degree do we believe that all instruction should be planned out in advance as part of the formal curriculum? To what degree do we tolerate, or even seek out opportunities for ad hoc learning, seizing the so-called teachable moments that arise over the course of the workday?

If we think that all learning should be highly programmed in advance, or if we are simply so busy clinically that we think we do not have time to teach while caring for patients, then teachable moments are likely to pass below our radar screen. On the other hand, if we think that lessons that arise out of daily practice are among the most memorable for learners, then we are likely to pause from time to time during the workday to make sure that we take advantage of important learning opportunities.

Determining what learners have learned is frequently referred to as assessment. Are the medical students doing a good job of learning what they most need to know? How can we tell? What is the best assessment technique? Is it written multiple-choice examinations? Is it interviews? Is it watching the students in action, demonstrating the knowledge and skills they have acquired in caring for patients, either simulated or actual? Again, whether we recognize it or not, our theories of learning are in play.

How does the assessment process look to learners? How useful do they find our assessments in improving their own learning performance? Which would be better: a single letter grade at the end of a month-long rotation, or weekly or even daily performance appraisals that include advice on how to do better? Do we see assessment as primarily summative, that is, providing an overview of how learners have done? Or do we see it in primarily formative terms, aimed at helping learners do a better job of learning? If our learning theory says that improving learning is more important than selecting and sorting learners, then our practice is likely to incline in the latter direction.

Consider a crude learning theory. Suppose we thought that learning is really just the pouring of information from full vessels (the educators) to empty vessels (the learners). On this theory, doing a better job educationally might mean pouring more information, and educators might aim to convey to students the greatest possible amount of information. Learning, on this view, is simply retaining what has been poured into you. The best way to teach is the one that enables you to convey the most information in the least amount of time. Reading assignments should be long, lectures are a good way to teach, and educational interactions should be modeled after data transmission.

How do we know whether learners are performing well? We open them up, metaphorically speaking, and see what spills out. That is, how much of what they have read and heard are they able to reproduce on an examination that tests recall? Although most of us would see some serious shortcomings in such a model, we might also acknowledge that it is not too far removed from the practice of some educators and institutions.

The first learning theory to be considered here is behaviorism. The great progenitor of behaviorist psychology was the Russian experimentalist Ivan Pavlov. Pavlov demonstrated that dogs that had initially not reacted to the sound of a bell but heard a bell ring each time they were fed learned to salivate at the sound of the bell, a process he called operant conditioning. The dog, in other words, had developed a new and reproducible behavior, salivation, in response to the stimulus of the bell.

Behaviorism developed in the early and mid-twentieth century as a reaction to psychological theories that were regarded as difficult to operationalize in empirical research methods. In an effort to develop an experimental approach to psychology and learning, early behaviorists such as John Watson developed the stimulus–response model. A stimulus is an externally administered sensory cue that might be visual, auditory, tactile, or even painful. A response is simply the subject's behavioral reaction. By manipulating stimuli appropriately, behaviorists thought, it is possible to achieve control of the subject's behavior. New behaviors might be learned, and old behaviors might be extinguished. Watson argued that the same conditioning that Pavlov had achieved with his dogs could be equally well applied to human beings. In the human case, additional stimuli and responses might be involved. For example, the stimulus might be praise, and the response might be correctly answering questions on a multiple-choice exam. Fundamentally, however, the stimulus–response model was the same. It did not matter what was going on inside the subject, in the case of learning theory, the mind of the student. What mattered was the subject's externally observable behavior.

The mind was a kind of black box, into which it was impossible to peer. In fact, it seemed doubtful to some behaviorists that the very notion of mind was meaningful. We should simply stop talking about minds, ideas, and emotions altogether, and instead focus on behavior. B.F. Skinner took this model even further, arguing that from a strict behaviorist perspective the very ideas of human freedom and dignity had become outmoded, and should be dispensed with (Fig. 2.1).

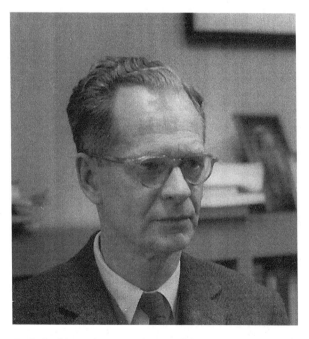

Fig. 2.1 Burrhus Frederic Skinner (1904–1990). One of the most influential psychologists of the twentieth century, Skinner's 21 books advanced radical behaviorism, the view that psychologists should focus on observable behaviors rather than hidden thoughts and emotions, and that reinforcements including rewards and punishments are the most important shapers of behavior. What would our accounts of education look like if we ruled out any reference to unobservable perceptions, thoughts, and emotions? Do great educators need to concern themselves with things they cannot directly observe? (Courtesy of Wikimedia Commons)

In the longstanding debate over whether nature or nurture exerted more influence over human character, the behaviorists were firmly on the side of nurture. As John Watson wrote: Give me a dozen healthy infants, well formed, and my own specified world to bring them up in, and I'll guarantee to take any one at random and train him to become any type of specialist I might select—doctor, lawyer, artist, merchant—regardless of his talents, penchants, tendencies, abilities, vocations, and race of his ancestors. Building on Darwinian biology, some behaviorists stressed the exigencies of biological existence in their accounts of what makes human beings tick. The learner, like every biological organism, exists fundamentally to survive. To a living being, survival comes first, and the most important stimuli for educators to focus on are those that pertain most directly to survival. What are our most basic biological needs? They include the needs for air, water, food, sleep, and relief from pain. To produce the greatest changes in learner behavior, educators should focus on such stimuli.

For example, if the only way learners can reduce painful stimuli such as electric shocks is by exhibiting a new behavior, they will quickly learn to exhibit that new behavior. Likewise, if access to food or water depends on a change in behavior, new behaviors are likely to be learned relatively quickly. What is learning? Change in behavior. What motivates behavior change? Stimuli. Thus, the educator is above all a manipulator of stimuli. When it comes to learning new behaviors, educators should avoid creating negative associations and seek to create positive associations.

The learner, then, is little more than a collection of stimulus–response associations. When new stimulus–response associations need to be created, as in the educational setting, there are only two types of responses. There are correct responses, and there are incorrect responses. The educator's mission is to withhold reward, or better yet punish the incorrect responses, and withhold punishment, or better yet reward, the correct responses. How do we know which responses are correct and which are incorrect? The answer is in the mind of the educator. Over time, a determined educator who brooks no opposition can engrain the correct responses and extinguish the incorrect responses.

From the behaviorist's point of view, the curriculum is little more than a set of behaviors that educators want to engrain in their learners. These behaviors might take the form of facts that can be recited or procedures that can be demonstrated. From the behaviorist's point of view, every learner is pretty much the same as every other learner. Their past experiences, knowledge, and habits do not matter, except insofar as they make it more or less easy to engrain new behaviors. Certainly, by the end of the educational experience, every learner should behave just like every other, reliably manifesting the desired behavior. What does instruction look like? Basically, the learners do what they are being told to do, or at least rewarded to do. The feedback learners receive should tell them in as straightforward a manner as possible whether they are responding correctly or incorrectly, rewarding the former and punishing the latter. In terms of assessment, behaviorists stress uniform procedures, such as standardized, written, multiple-choice exams. The difference between correct and incorrect responses is obvious, and performance is easily scored. If a learner is not performing well, you simply lean on them harder until they get it.

The next learning theory is gestalt psychology. Gestalt psychology is frequently associated with optical illusions, images that can be interpreted in two or more very different ways. Examples include well-known paintings that can be interpreted as a vase or two faces looking at each other, or the line drawing that can be interpreted as a young woman looking away from the viewer or an old woman looking to the side of the viewer. *Gestalt* is a German word that denotes shape or form, and one of the key ideas behind gestalt psychology is the view that a set of sensory stimuli can be interpreted in different ways, or remain fundamentally incoherent, depending on what is happening in the mind of the observer.

Unlike the behaviorists, the gestalt psychologists believed that it is vital to attempt to peer inside the mind of the learner, to see how we find or create meaning in the world around us. Examples of the construction of more complex orders of meaning from simpler components include a motion picture, where the eye sees a rapid sequence of static images that the mind assembles into a continuous sequence of motion. Other examples include our perception of constellations among the stars, melodies from successions of notes, and medical diagnoses from collections of symptoms, signs, physical exam findings, laboratory results, and so on.

The gestalt psychologists sought to identify rules by which we find order in the world around us. In terms of visual experience, one key rule is similarity. We are more likely to see coherent order where visual objects are relatively alike in terms of size, color, shape, and so on. Proximity is likewise important. If objects are close to one another, we are more likely to see them as belonging together in some way. In the case of music, if the notes are separated too much from one another in time, we may not discern a coherent melody, but only a series of disconnected tones.

Continuity is also important. If we can establish a series or sequence, then an object's boundaries will likely appear to lie where that sequence is broken. For example, we might turn one row of dots into two rows of dots, simply by removing the middle dot.

Finally, there is the principle of closure, which says that we have a natural tendency to see limits to things. For example, even if there is a small gap in a circle, we are still likely to see it as a circle, because doing so brings it to a kind of perceptual closure. Likewise, it can be difficult to detect certain spelling errors, because our mind tends to correct them before they reach consciousness.

In education, gestalt psychology emphasizes problem solving. The behaviorists are largely interested in learners' abilities to repeat something they have seen or done, but the gestalt psychologist especially prizes the ability to solve problems in novel situations. In the nonhuman sphere, an example is that of an ape placed on a ledge separated from another ledge by a chasm too wide to traverse. On the other side is food. How can the ape get the food? Apes have been observed to solve the problem by using a stick to reach across the chasm and retrieve the food.

In the human sphere, oncologists sought some means to deliver a lethal dose of radiation to a tumor in the center of the brain without damaging the surrounding normal parenchyma. How could they do it? A brilliant inspiration was the idea of using two or three lower-dose beams that converged only at the site of the tumor, where a lethal dose was delivered. In both cases, the learner has a sort of "Aha!" experience, where the solution to a puzzle emerges in a new form or pattern.

How would a gestalt psychologist tend to approach curriculum, instruction, and assessment? First, the curriculum would consist less of facts or techniques that learners are simply expected to memorize and more of problems that learners are expected to solve. The goal is to foster the ability to solve novel problems. The aim is not so much to challenge learners' mental storage capacities as their ability to improvise and invent, perceiving new distinctions and connections where none were apparent before. The emphasis is on creating new and meaningful wholes. How is that possible instructionally? It is important to challenge learners to organize and reorganize their knowledge. Learning tasks should invite them to examine their most basic assumptions in the search for new ways of putting together what is before them. Knowledge is not a collection of facts, but an array of habits by which to examine the world from multiple perspectives. Assessment is less focused on regurgitation and more focused on problem solving and creativity. The assessment becomes a kind of learning experience in itself.

Cognitive psychology is similar to gestalt psychology in that both stress the development of meaning from experience. In cognitive psychology, however, greater stress is placed on the idea of information processing. Particularly, as computer science has developed, cognitive psychologists have tended to employ models drawn from computers for understanding what goes on in the minds of learners. Cognitive psychologists developed one of the most widely accepted models of how the memory functions.

In one widely discussed model, the memory consists of three principal parts, the sensory registers, short-term memory, and long-term memory. To an educator, the sensory registers are important because learners cannot retain what they do not notice. Thus, educators need to make their material appealing to the senses. Short-term memory is important because learners may be able to retain facts in short-term memory long enough to reproduce them on a test, but not really retain them. The real goal of education is to implant ideas in long-term memory, so that learners can use them throughout their lives.

More perhaps than gestalt psychology, cognitive psychology seeks to open up the black box of the mind and discern how information is processed by it. One way to do this is to ask learners to speak out loud or otherwise record what they are thinking. Again, the focus is less on merely repeating what has been seen or heard than on solving problems. Responses are not simply right or wrong, they are also important clues to what the learner is thinking. Incorrect responses can be even more revealing than correct ones in helping educators to better understand the mind of the learner.

Rather than simply classifying responses as correct or incorrect, we should be asking ourselves this question: what are we learning about how the learner is approaching this problem, and how could we use that knowledge to improve problem solving in the future? Memory is important, but so is creativity, and the learner's own ability to learn from failures. Another important capacity to foster is metacognition, learners' awareness of and insight into their own learning. Are they not only learning but learning about learning, and can they put that learning to use to learn better?

From an educational point of view, cognitive psychology prizes curriculum that not only conveys information but helps learners become better problem solvers and develop their own metacognitive abilities. Learning activities should foster the self-awareness of learners. Educators should determine what separates novices from experts and help learners to make that transition as effectively and efficiently as possible. It is not only what experts know in the sense of facts, but how they do what they do. When showed a game in progress, a chess expert instantly recognizes where the strategic advantage lies.

Similarly, expert physicians can often see the diagnosis very quickly, whereas novices may never arrive at it. Instruction involves helping novices see the minds of experts at work, observing not only what they say but how they arrive at their impressions. In terms of assessment, learners should be presented with challenges that require them to try out different strategies. Which cognitive map best matches this particular terrain? And what can we do to help learners become more self-aware?

Constructivism is associated with the work of pioneers such as John Dewey and Lev Vygotsky. Behaviorism, gestalt psychology, and cognitivist approaches all tend to focus on individual learners, but, constructivism emphasizes the social dimension of learning. In the late twentieth century, constructivists became disenchanted with the computer as a model of the human mind. They believed that information cannot be properly understood apart from the social situations in which it is embedded. There is no such thing as decontextualized information or skills. Instead, what we know and what we can do are powerfully influenced by culture.

Constructivism takes its name from the view that knowledge is not really discovered at all, but rather constructed by human beings. What we know is the product of two highly interrelated factors, the nature of the known and the nature of the knower, which can never be completely disentangled from each other. Hence, we need to focus on what is going on in the minds of learners, and in particular, among learners. Learning is not an individual sport but a team sport.

Different constructivists have viewed learning in different ways. Some take a largely rational view of learning, and suggest that educators and learners should be seen as engaged in a process of systematic inquiry that is governed by objectively established methodological rules. Others take a more sociopolitical view of learning, arguing that all rules are themselves social constructions, and there are no objective standards to which educators can appeal. From this point of view, learning is often regarded in terms of power relations, where powerful teachers attempt to impose their views on their relatively weak and impressionable students.

From both points of view, however, the knower and the learning environment are inseparable. The educator's task is to support inquiry on the part of learners, helping them to collaborate with one another as they develop their own understanding of the subject matter. The collaborative approach applies to educators and students as well, who become coinvestigators and cocreators of meaning. The constructivist approach places special emphasis on challenging learners as members of groups, rather than as individuals.

From the constructivist point of view, curriculum is not a received body of knowledge but a set of challenges to which learners should respond. The educator's mission is to present them with the sorts of problems they will confront in real-life practice in their field. Knowledge does not flow from educators to learners, but is developed collaboratively when the two are encouraged to work together. There is no single fixed body of knowledge that every learner must acquire, and the best educators can do is to prepare learners to continue to learn for themselves.

Instructionally, learners are not recipients of information, but active explorers of the field. Learning is an adventure, and missteps and failures are an inevitable and even desirable part of the learning process, as long as they are seized upon as learning opportunities. It is more difficult to separate instruction and assessment, inasmuch as both are going on simultaneously in the best learning environments. We cannot compare learners' performance to some prescribed answer key, but must instead watch learners in action.

Each of these four learning has strengths and weaknesses, and none is perfect by itself. By deepening our understanding of what takes place in the minds of learners, we can enhance our educational effectiveness.

Expertise

In thinking about how to educate physicians, it is important to consider the end product we hope to produce. What is our vision of a well-educated physician? What would it mean to excel as a physician, and how can we best prepare medical students and residents to attain that level of performance? It is unrealistic to expect new graduates to function at the same level as physicians with decades of experience, but it would be a mistake not to launch them on a trajectory that leads to genuine expertise. First-rate physicians are not merely competent, they are experts, and we should prepare our trainees to achieve this level of excellence. In order to prepare them to function as experts, however, we must first understand what it means to be an expert. What distinguishes experts from novices, and what does it take to move from mere competence to expertise?

The word expert is drawn from the Latin root *experientia*, which means proof, trial, or experiment. An expert is someone who has attained a high level of understanding or proficiency as a result of a great deal of experience, and is recognized as a resource to whom other people should turn for advice. A novice, by contrast, is someone who has little or no experience. Drawn from the same Latin root as our word novel, a novice is literally new at some field of endeavor, like a medical student or resident on the first day of training. Competence comes from the Latin root *competere*, which means to be capable or qualified. Before novices can become experts, they must first become competent, and many of us become competent at particular tasks or fields of endeavor without ever becoming truly expert.

If we are serious about promoting expertise, genuine excellence as opposed to mere competence, then we must distinguish between two different types of educational outcomes, processes and performances. One means of academic and professional credentialing is based on processes. How many years of training has an individual completed? Where did the training take place, who were the instructors, and what enrichment opportunities were provided? Has he or she passed the requisite examinations? Such credentials provide important information about a physician, but they do not themselves prove that the individual performs well in practice. To know professionals' level of excellence in practice, we need to observe them in practice. Frequently, if we are to make a high-quality assessment, we need an expert to do the observing.

What makes an expert truly expert? To say simply that experts are the people in a group who perform best at particular tasks is to beg the question. It is similarly unhelpful to say that experts simply know more than everyone else. Expertise is not the mere accretion of facts, nor is it merely repeated practice. Knowledge and skills can be inert. The expert not only knows a lot and can perform some tasks very well, the expert can use that knowledge and those skills to successfully negotiate new challenges. It is not merely that the expert sees all the pieces of the puzzle. The expert can see how those pieces fit together, and perhaps even combine and recombine them in novel and productive ways. The expert functions at a higher level of imaginative integration, seeing important patterns that others miss.

This higher level of integration enables the expert to perform tasks more quickly. A merely competent practitioner may have to go through a whole mental checklist, or may require hours or even days to perceive a pattern that is apparent to the expert almost instantly. In some cases, the pattern is visible only to the expert. The expert knows what is most important in a particular picture, and focuses right away on those features, whether it be a constellation of signs and symptoms or a collection of experimental results. It is not only that the expert knows the answers, but the expert knows what questions to ask. An expert radiologist knows how to interrogate a CT scan to extract the relevant information effectively and efficiently. To the expert's eye, some features are simply more interesting—that is, they offer a higher cognitive yield—than others.

The expert's ability stems in part from what cognitive psychologists have called chunking. Chunking is the ability to group multiple data together under a single coherent rubric. A novice looking at the starry night sky sees innumerable randomly situated points of light. When experts look at the same thing, they see numerous constellations, and can instantly call to mind the astronomical properties of the different stars they see. The operation of memory provides a well-known example of chunking. Most of us would have great difficulty recalling a string of 28 random numbers. If, however, those numbers happen to represent a sequence of the four phone numbers we dial most frequently, then they may become quite easy to recall. Experts are able to organize their perception and thinking in such a way that they can process large collections of information as coherent chunks.

When novices look at a patient, they do not know where to begin. What is germane to the diagnostic task at hand, and what is irrelevant? What represents a mere distractor, such as the vehicle that brought the patient to the hospital, and what is a vital bit of information, such as what the patient was doing when the symptoms began? Experts can often tell in a split second whether a particular finding is normal or abnormal, because they hone in instantly on the key distinguishing features. It is not just that they have seen dozens or hundreds or thousands of such cases, but that they have learned from those experiences to focus their attention on the features with the highest diagnostic yield. They are not merely experienced practitioners, but reflective practitioners, who have thoroughly mined their clinical experience for whatever lessons it can offer. From an educational point of view, the crucial question is whether expertise can be shared with learners, and if so, how to do it.

It is possible that there are no real shortcuts to expertise. To become a truly world-class chess player, for example, may require something on the order of 50,000 h of chess playing (Fig. 2.2). No one can sit down with a book about chess, or attend chess classes, and become an expert in several hundred or several thousand hours. Perhaps even more significant is the realization that expertise tends to be highly domain specific. Just because people become experts at chess does not mean that they will be expert mathematicians, linguists, or psychologists. Similarly, a physician who is an expert in cardiology may not perform better than average in another discipline, such as gastroenterology. Likewise, expert physicians are not necessarily good leaders, managers, or businesspeople.

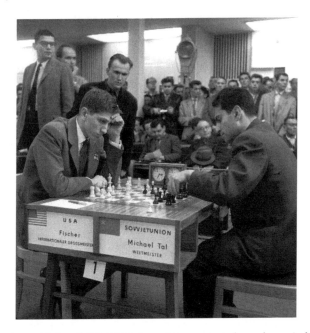

Fig. 2.2 Robert James Fischer (1943–2008). One of the greatest chess players in history, Bobby Fischer first encountered chess at the age of 6. He became obsessed with the game, devoting most of his waking life to playing and reading about chess, and winning his first US championship as a 14 year old. He is pictured here playing the reigning world champion in Leipzig at the age of 17. Some experts estimate that the development of true expertise requires approximately 10 years or 10,000 h of dedicated practice (Courtesy of Wikimedia)

Chess offers another interesting insight into expertise. It turns out that a world-class chess player can absorb a great deal of information about a chess match in a very short period of time. Shown a particular chess game in progress, an expert can often reproduce the position of most or all the pieces on the board after looking at it for only a second or so. By contrast, a novice might have great difficulty reproducing the position of more than a few pieces. However, the expert's ability is limited in a particularly revealing way. Experts can only reproduce the position of the pieces when their position represents an actual game of chess. If the pieces are randomly positioned, the expert performs little better than the novice. This indicates that expertise requires meaning. That is, the expert must understand the pieces as fitting into some larger strategic configuration if their position is to be memorable.

How could we capitalize on these insights in medical education? First, we need to focus our educational efforts in ways that highlight integrating concepts. Our aim is not to download reams of data, but to help learners locate and begin to exploit approaches that bring order to what they will see in daily practice as clinicians, scientists, and educators. Although it is important to give learners an overview of the terrain in which they will be working, we sometimes err on the side of excessive breadth, at the expense of adequate depth. There are some things that future physicians merely need to know about, and others that they genuinely need to know well. Among the latter are organizing concepts, and especially concepts with leverage, that can be put to use in many different novel situations.

When lecturing, good introductory overviews can be invaluable. What are we going to talk about here? What are the key concepts that we hope to take away from this discussion? How might these concepts prove useful in daily practice? We cannot simply transfer such concepts into the minds of learners and expect them to begin using them productively, but we can provide them problems to work on and guidance about how to get started. We can provide valuable guidance by working on the problems ourselves, and doing so "out loud," so learners can see how we approach them. Confronted with a welter of data, how does an expert set to work? What sorts of questions help to get the ball rolling? What sorts of questions prove most helpful when you get stuck? How do you avoid latching onto the first idea that comes to mind, thereby truncating the search for even better ones?

One powerful element of medical expertise is a thorough understanding of pathophysiology. A variety of seemingly disparate and unconnected symptoms, signs, physical examination findings, and laboratory results may fit together very nicely once we understand their common basis in pathophysiology. The expert is able to use extensive pathophysiological understanding to sift from a huge body of knowledge the particular ideas that are most likely to be relevant to the case at hand. None of us ever use everything we know to solve a problem, and one of the first tasks in solving any problem is to determine which of our prior experiences offer insight. The novice must thumb through a large reference work page by page, looking for a similar example, whereas the expert is able to turn quickly to the relevant section. The expert's understanding may be likened to a handy index that organizes a much larger text.

If we take this lesson seriously, we should ensure that our evaluations of learners reflect this principle. Exams should not merely test the ability to recall specific facts, but to organize facts in larger contexts. As long as knowledge remains at the level of individual facts, it is inert. To bring it to life, we must invite learners to use that knowledge in solving problems. Suppose a patient presents with hematuria, blood in the urine. We should not merely ask for a laundry list of pathological processes that may cause hematuria. We should invite learners to begin developing ordered diagnostic hypotheses based on their understanding of pathophysiology and the facts of the particular case at hand. For example, is the bleeding painful or painless? Does the patient have an abdominal mass? Are there bacteria in the patient's urine? By using case scenarios to assess learner understanding, we encourage learners to think in ways that will serve them best in caring for patients.

Experts not only get the right answers. They also look for better questions. When a novice asks a question of an expert, the expert may do more for the novice by asking a question than by providing the answer. For example, the novice may present a choice between two different options for diagnostic testing, but the expert may, by asking a question of the novice, point out that additional history taking might render both tests unnecessary. Our ideal of expertise should not be a person who knows all the answers. Our vision should be someone who is able to pose and recognize good questions, and who knows how to go about finding out the answers. We need to foster a certain skepticism among our trainees, so that they eventually ask better questions than we have managed to ask. The future advance of medical knowledge depends on such inquisitiveness.

We should also bear in mind that expertise has its limitations. In some cases, expertise can serve as much as a barrier as a springboard. For example, experts do not always make good teachers. An expert may understand a subject so well that it is difficult to appreciate what it looks like to novices. The expert may know where the learners should be headed, but find it very difficult to discern where they are, and thus experience difficulty moving them from point A to point B. In some cases, merely competent individuals may make better educators, because they can better understand and relate to the people they are teaching. In some cases, residents may make better teachers than faculty members, and medical students may make better teachers than residents. This is not to say that experts cannot understand learners better than anyone, but only that they do not always do so.

For one thing, expertise in education itself can be quite valuable in the development of educational excellence. People who understand learning may be better equipped to teach than people who do not. The same might go for curriculum design, the development of new instructional techniques, and the assessment of learning. Although medical education clearly enjoys the services of many people who seem to be born educators, it is likely that everyone, even the best among us, could do a better job of teaching if we knew more about our students and how they learn. For those of us who are not naturally effective educators, such lessons might prove especially valuable.

We must also guard against the temptation to regard expertise in a close-minded way that stunts further investigation and learning. Having an expert in our midst should not make the rest of us lazier. Instead, it should act as a stimulus to further improvement for us all. The expert should not push us out of the way as though we were irrelevant, but challenge us to grow and develop. The goal is not to avoid getting caught having to admit that we do not know something, but seeking out the things we do not know and investigating them. Lack of understanding, unless it is the result of incuriosity or indolence, is not a sign of weakness, but an opportunity for learning. We should encourage our learners not to cover up what they do not know, but to grab it by the tail and follow it where it leads.

If being an expert means simply having all the answers, then the search for new understanding will inevitably be seen as a sign of weakness. Somebody who has to go looking for an answer must not have them all. In fact, however, we must first recognize that we do not know before we go looking for new knowledge. An expert is not someone who has stopped learning, but someone who learns every day. One of the most characteristic features of a physician expert is the habit of learning. The moment we stop learning is the moment we begin to become extinct. Moreover, learning is one of the most fulfilling aspects of a professional career, because learning is intrinsically enjoyable and enables us to do our jobs better.

Memory

Memory failures are universal. We bump into an old acquaintance, proceed to introduce the person to a companion, and then suddenly realize to our horror that we cannot recall the acquaintance's name. Or checking in for a flight at the airport to depart for a long-awaited vacation, we make the disheartening discovery that we left the passports at home. Or, about to offer a brilliant diagnostic opinion on a difficult clinical case, we discover that we cannot call to mind the name of a disease that we have dealt with on dozens of occasions. Such memory lapses are a familiar feature of the human experience. And it is their very familiarity that leads many of us not to devote to them the attention that they deserve. We simply take them for granted, like rainy days. As a result, many of us do not grasp the true complexity of memory and the many ways it can fail.

Few people need a rich and nuanced understanding of memory more than physicians. We use memory to detect findings, offer differential diagnoses, and arrive at recommendations for further evaluation and treatment. If our memory fails us, it can lead us to overlook a finding or to point out a finding when none is, in fact, present. It can cause us to offer incomplete or inaccurate diagnostic hypotheses. It may even lead us to draw mistaken conclusions from our own observations and hypotheses, resulting in harm to the patients for whom we care. To avoid such pitfalls and enable future physicians to do the same, we need to study memory with the same curiosity and dedication we bring to the practice and teaching of medicine. Our memory is at least as important a professional resource as our facilities and equipment. In some respects, in fact, memory is even more important, since none of our professional activities would be possible without it, and the quality of our all work hinges very much on the reliability of memory.

In his 2002 book, *The Seven Sins of Memory: How the Mind Forgets and Remembers*, Harvard University Psychologist Daniel Schacter discusses seven stereotypical ways in which memory can fail us. The discussion is premised on the view that if we better understand how memory lets us down, we can better protect against lapses and reduce the frequency and severity of adverse consequences. As a highly cognitive field requiring a high level of mnemonic performance, medicine needs to understand these patterns of failure and the steps we can take to counteract them. The point of briefly reviewing each of Schacter's categories of memory failure is not to suggest that they provide us with a final and infallible list of all errors mnemonic, but to begin to trace out the complexity of the subject.

Before reviewing each of the seven ways memory can fail us, it is important to highlight some categorical differences between them. The first group of three includes what we commonly call forgetting, the different ways in which we can fail to recall something. These are transience, absent mindedness, and blocking. Yet these are not the only ways in which memory can let us down, and the next group of three consists of failures not of forgetting but of remembering. Memory can cause just as much trouble when it leads us to recall something incorrectly as it does when we fail in our efforts to bring it to mind. These are misattribution, suggestibility, and bias. The final of the seven failures of memory belongs to still another category, namely, situations where we would like to forget something but are unable to do so. This is persistence.

The first failure of memory is the most familiar, transience. This refers to the general tendency for memories to diminish over time, such that more distant ideas and events are typically more difficult to call to mind than more recent ones. The adage, "Use it or lose it," applies no less to memory than to physical conditioning. Happily, however, such material can sometimes be relearned more quickly and easily than when it was first acquired. Hence, the value of "refresher" courses, which tend to operate on the assumption that we have seen the material before.

It is important to recognize that memory does not decay at a constant rate over time. Generally speaking, decay is relatively rapid in the near term, and then slows down. In other words, forgetting is a nonlinear process, a rule that holds for a wide variety of different cognitive settings. Moreover, forgetting is not all bad. It would be a curse to remember everything, because then our memories would be clogged with so much trivial and irrelevant information that it would be more difficult to call to mind what really matters. We select what is worth remembering by many means.

One way of enhancing the recall of learners is to highlight upcoming information as important. One means of doing this is to ask learners questions about a topic before introducing new information. Another is to make it clear to learners how new information will prove useful in the future. For example, an educator preparing to teach about adverse reactions to cardiopulmonary resuscitation might first present a scenario in which a patient collapses, and then ask learners how they would handle it. Simply getting learners to admit that they do not know and recognizing the magnitude of the potential consequences can make the material more memorable.

The next type of memory failure is absent mindedness. This refers to situations in which we intend to do something but fail to remember to do so. A memorable example involved the cellist Yo-Yo Ma, who was traveling by taxi to a performance. When he arrived at his destination, he suddenly realized that he had left his cello, valued at $2.5 million, in the cab. Had a hypothetical bystander asked him at any point where his cello was located, he would have immediately recalled that it was in the trunk of the cab, but because he was thinking about other things when he arrived at his destination, he failed to remember it. Such lapses tend to occur when we are operating on "auto pilot" and do not receive a cue we normally rely on to carry out a particular action. The difficulty is not so much failing to bring to mind something we are searching for, but rather failing to search in the first place.

Such lapses can befall any physician. Interruptions in our normal routine can deprive us of clues we normally rely on to recall certain tasks. Such failures can be hazardous, in part because, by definition, we do not even recognize that they are occurring. This is one reason that healthcare organizations have been adopting "time out" policies to ensure that teams verify basic assumptions (Correct patient? Correct site? Correct dose?) before administering medications and performing procedures. We cannot teach learners to remember everything, but by encouraging them to identify high-stakes situations and put in place systems to detect and compensate for occasional lapses, we can help them reduce the frequency and magnitude of costly errors.

The third memory lapse is blocking. Though blocking might seem identical to transience, the two are in fact very different. When a memory is blocked, it is not merely unavailable, it is also actively screened out by other memories. We have not completely forgotten the information, but have temporarily lost access to it. We may be able to recall something similar to what we are seeking, but the sought-after item does not come to mind. For example, a physician might be able to recall many features of a particular disease, such as Langerhans cell histiocytosis, including its different types and varied manifestations, yet fail to recall its name. Sometime later—whether 5 min, 5 h, or 5 days—the sought-after information effortlessly comes to mind. The difficulty in this situation seems to lie in search and retrieval, a mismatch between what we are looking for and how we are looking for it.

Blocking is so familiar that many different human languages have a phrase that corresponds to having a word "on the tip of the tongue." It represents an active process, at least to the extent that we can think of words or phrases like the one we are searching for, and make determinations about whether or not we have found the right one. Somewhere in the mind is a judge who knows whether we have come up with the word we are looking for. At times it seems that we have caught hold of it for a second, but then, inexplicably, it slips away. Generally, we experience a small sense of victory and relief when we finally find the right word or it finds us. Such lapses sometimes occur at embarrassing moments, but we can take some comfort in the fact that the people we are speaking with have undoubtedly experienced the same thing. By helping learners develop the habit of attempting to access such information from multiple points of view, employ effective electronic search strategies, and sometimes just wait patiently for its return, we can help them deal more effectively with blocked items.

The next category of memory lapses concerns situations where a memory is present but wrong. In other words, this is a form of memory distortion. The first of these is misattribution. This occurs when we remember something, but we ascribe it to an incorrect source. Consider, for example, the misidentification of a suspect in a criminal case. A witness saw or heard something, but attributes it to the wrong person, with potentially devastating legal consequences. This phenomenon can also lead to serious problems in medicine. For example, a physician may misattribute a doubtful idea to a highly reputable and trustworthy source, promoting an unwarranted level of reliance on it when closer inspection is indicated. Another example of misattribution would be thinking that we did something when we in fact did not, because we imagine ourselves having done it. In such a case, we attribute to memory something that in fact occurred only in the imagination.

In short, misattribution can lead us to remember things that never happened. Consider the following well-known and reproducible example of this phenomenon. If someone recites a list of words including candy, sour, sugar, bitter, taste, cake, eat, pie, and so on, and then asks us whether the word taste was on the list, most of us will say correctly that it was. However, if we are asked if the word sweet was on the list, we will likely say yes again, even though it was not. The mind is not a mere transcriptionist, taking down and reading back what we say and hear. Instead it also finds meaning in experiences. When all of the words on a list we are being asked to recall belong to a category that would include the word sweet, we think we heard it.

Something similar can happen in medical reasoning, when a constellation of findings points strongly to a particular diagnosis, and soon we find ourselves accepting the diagnosis without sufficiently exploring the counterevidence and evidence in favor of other diagnostic possibilities. This phenomenon is sometimes referred to as premature closure, a phenomenon that becomes more common as we age, and therefore represents a form of memory lapse against which more mature radiologists should be particularly aware of. We can help learners to avoid such pitfalls by encouraging them to develop the habit of stepping back and reexamining hypotheses from alternative points of view.

Suggestibility refers to the proclivity of questions and manners of questioning to shape the answers we offer. Consider the following demonstration: "What color is snow? What color are clouds? What color is a bride's gown? What do cows drink?" Most people will respond milk, even though the correct answer would be water, because the preceding questions have prepared us to respond with something associated with the color white. In a court room proceeding, questions can be posed in a leading fashion that tends to suggest a certain answer, independent of whether the suggested answer is correct. This form of memory lapse has precipitated grave consequences in legal cases concerning trauma and abuse, where witnesses have recalled events that never happened or happened quite differently from what they recall. The way in which questions are posed can particularly powerfully influence what children do and do not seem to recall.

An example of this pitfall in medicine concerns clinical history. Absent or erroneous clinical history can lead a physician to over- or underestimate the true probability of a particular diagnosis. For example, if a clinical history of immunodeficiency is omitted, the physician may fail to consider the possibility that respiratory symptoms and signs may represent opportunistic infection. On the other hand, a clinical history of infection may lead to the assumption that bone pain is due to infection, when in fact it is a malignancy such as a Ewing sarcoma.

Medical learners need to be mindful of suggestibility. One way of counteracting it is to make sure to review records thoroughly, thereby ensuring that other important information is not omitted from the discussion. Another means is to be sure to look and think for oneself, not simply relying on the reported observations and conclusions of others. It is vital both prospectively and retrospectively to avoid allowing the way a clinical question is presented to preclude additional and potentially more momentous observations that a colleague may have discounted or failed to consider all together.

The next type of memory error is bias. This involves the tendency for more recent knowledge and beliefs to distort our recollection of others situated in the more distant past. For example, physicians' general assessment of the intensity and stress of after-hours on-call duties may be especially strongly influenced by their last few on-call shifts. If those shifts proved to be particularly demanding, they may regard on-call duties, in general, as more strenuous than had their few most recent shifts been light. This phenomenon reminds us again that the human memory is not merely a data storage device like a voice recorder. Instead interpretation is taking place at every step of the "storage" and "retrieval" processes, and our memory (or lack thereof) for any event or idea is powerfully affected by the meaning we attribute to it.

In clinical practice, one common manifestation of bias is to consider more strongly diagnoses that we have recently encountered in clinical practice, sometimes referred to as recency bias. We ask ourselves, "What has turned out to be the diagnosis in patients who presented similarly in the past?" but all cases that come to mind are not recalled with equal prominence. The recent cases are generally more memorable, or at least more likely to influence diagnostic reasoning. As a result, we may place too much emphasis on what we have seen recently, and overlook less immediately familiar but nonetheless important diagnostic possibilities. To guard against such bias, we need to make learners aware of this bias and encourage them to assess probabilities based on large case series that do not rely solely on the memory of any particular individual.

The final form of memory failure, which differs from the other six, is persistence. This refers to the unwanted recollection of things that we would prefer to forget. For example, a physician who has been named in a malpractice suit may be haunted by memories of the experience long after the matter has been resolved, even if it was decided in the physician's favor. This phenomenon lies behind what has been called "post-traumatic stress disorder," where well-intentioned efforts to help victims "process" and "work through" difficult experiences have sometimes made it even more difficult for them to put the experience behind them and move on. Less dramatically, some physicians who have made an error may be so preoccupied by it that they find it difficult to concentrate on other work for the rest of the day.

All unpleasant memories should not be forgotten. To recall only the pleasant experiences of life would be to leave out an important part of the story, and thereby prevent the discovery of important lessons. Making mistakes is no fun, but every mistake is also a learning opportunity, and it is important that we recognize errors, explore them, and attempt to apply lessons learned to improve future performance. Often, at least a portion of each intrusive memory is related less to the actual event itself than to the way we interpret it. By encouraging learners to talk about the experience with a counselor, colleague, or friend, it is often possible to help them see the experience in a new light that makes it both less threatening and easier to live with. Merely discussing such memories with someone else can often prove therapeutic in itself.

It would be tempting to suppose that a "perfect" memory would be a blessing. Recent media reports have described several individuals with "hyperthymestic syndrome," a kind of super memory. One such individual, sometimes described as the "person who could not forget," is a middle-aged woman who is able to reproduce highly detailed accounts of every day of her life since she was 14 years old. In fact, however, her memory is only out of the ordinary when it comes to recalling autobiographical details, and she lacks any extraordinary ability to recall facts that do not pertain to her own life. Her condition may be less a manifestation of exceptional memory than an extreme form of obsessive-compulsive disorder, centered around her own life and past.

As this case reminds us, mnemonic performance is a much more complex matter than merely whether or not we are able to recall a particular item. The inability to bring something to mind has multiple possible causes. Likewise, the mere fact that we are able to recall an idea does not necessarily imply that we have recalled it correctly or that our lives are going to be enriched by retaining it. By helping learners to explore memory more deeply and apply an understanding of its stereotypical forms of failure to their professional and personal lives, we can help them recall what is most worth remembering, avoid the pitfall of supposing they know something when they really do not, and prevent intrusive memories from undermining the quality of their lives.

Concepts of Health and Disease

At the core of medicine lie the concepts of health and disease. Medicine aims to cure disease, or at least relieve the suffering related to it, and where possible, to prevent it from arising. Moreover, health promotion is increasingly recognized as an important part of the physician's mission, so that people can lead lives as full and rich as possible. Yet the concepts of health and disease are not so simple and straightforward as we might first suppose. For example, do we distinguish between a person who is merely feeling badly and a person who is really sick? Do physicians and hospitals bear responsibility for treating every form of human suffering? Is health a mere absence of disease and injury, or is it a positive state of well-being? If today's medical students and residents are to achieve their full potential as physicians, it is important that they base their practice on a complete and rich vision of what it means to be healthy.

Let us suppose that a patient presents to a physician's office complaining of not feeling well. How do we determine whether patients are sick, and if so, what ails them? One approach would be to obtain sophisticated diagnostic tests on the blood, or to order radiological studies in order to glimpse the anatomy and physiology of the patient's internal organs. In most cases, however, such sophisticated diagnostic studies are not indicated, and the history alone or the history and the physical examination provide more than adequate diagnostic information. Despite the fact that more sophisticated diagnostic studies are usually unneeded, they shape our vision of medical practice to an ever-greater degree. For example, some patients who present with headaches may feel cheated if their physician does not order a computed tomography (CT) scan to ensure that they do not have a brain tumor. Likewise, physicians may feel that we are not doing our best for our patients if we do not avail ourselves of medicine's full diagnostic armamentarium.

We need to understand more deeply what it means to be ill, and to clarify our vision of the state of health in which we seek to enable our patients to live. The World Health Organization's Second International Classification of Functioning, Disability, and Health (ICIDH-2) provides a useful point of departure in this regard. As modified here, it approaches health and disease in terms of four levels or tiers: structure, function, activity, and participation. The underlying presumption is that health and disease cannot be adequately understood on any single level, and a multitiered approach is necessary. Like the molecular, cellular, organic, organismal, and communal approaches to understanding living organisms, we need to look from multiple different angles if we aim to understand fully the impact of illness on a patient's life.

The most basic level of health and disease is structure. This is the traditional forte of the anatomist, the pathologist, the surgeon, and the radiologist. In order to discern what is wrong with a patient, we must discover what portion of their structure is out of shape. To know whether someone is ill, we seek a structural abnormality. If the appendix has a normal appearance, with no trace of inflammation, then we dismiss the diagnosis of appendicitis. If a patient with cough and fever has a normal chest radiograph, we know that they do not have pneumonia, although they could have a raging case of bronchitis. If a febrile patient has a normal white blood cell count and blood smear, we know that bacterial infection is not the culprit. When a patient presents with abdominal pain, we work our way through the organs of the belly until we find one that accounts for the patient's symptoms.

In so doing, we are continually weighing the appearance of the patient's anatomy against that of our mental image of normalcy. The crucial determination we are always trying to make is both stunningly simple and mind-bogglingly complex: is this normal or abnormal? If the finding is within the range of normal, we dismiss it. If we suspect that it is abnormal, we set about attempting to determine what it might be. We formulate a differential diagnosis, and then take additional steps to sort out which option is most probable. In some cases, we arrive at a definitive diagnosis, as when a bone radiograph clearly reveals a fracture. In other cases, we never know for sure what the matter with the patient was, or even whether the patient was really sick to begin with. Yet where the structural tier of health and disease is concerned, it is worth remembering that even a completely normal diagnostic test does not definitively rule out the possibility of disease. The bone radiograph may be initially normal, and it is only a week later, after demineralization has taken place and some periosteal reaction has formed adjacent to the fracture that we are able to recognize a nondisplaced hairline fracture. Even our most sophisticated imaging studies may not show us the pathology. For example, a patient with severe psychosis may have a normal magnetic resonance imaging (MRI) exam of the brain. Conversely, there is no guarantee that every patient with an abnormality of diagnostic testing actually has the disease. A solitary pulmonary nodule may represent a granuloma, and not a lung cancer at all.

We need to recall that no diagnostic test is 100% accurate, and the accuracy of every test varies depending on the circumstances in which it is used. We can generate costly false positives by employing a test in circumstances where the initial probability of disease is very low. If medicine is to provide optimal value to patients and our communities, it is important that we educate future physicians to understand not only how to interpret diagnostic tests, but when to use and when not to use them. It is a mistake to suppose that the quality of medical care is directly proportional to the number of tests the physician orders. In many situations, the best test is no test at all. If learners are to understand how to employ diagnostic testing effectively, they need to recognize that ferreting out abnormal structures is not the highest objective of medicine.

The second tier of health and disease is function. To understand function, we must look beyond the snapshots of the structural tier and think of health and disease as unfolding in time. The coronal, sagittal, and axial dimensions do not tell the whole story. We must see how they are changing from minute to minute, day to day, and year to year. It is not enough to know that there is a hole in the heart. It is necessary to know what that hole means to the function of the cardiovascular system. Is it permitting too much deoxygenated blood to enter into the systemic circulation? Is it jamming the lungs with too much blood, and thereby making the heart work too hard to supply an adequate amount of blood to the brain, heart, and kidneys? To know what a structural abnormality really amounts to, we must understand its functional implications.

Although the functional level of understanding cannot simply supplant the structural level, it does enjoy a higher level of explanatory power. We can suffer structural insults of one kind or another, yet through functional redundancy or retraining, return to our formal level of function. For example, some patients recover virtually completely from a stroke, despite the fact that they have suffered the irreversible loss of a portion of their brain tissue. The dominance of function over structure is apparent in the design of prosthetic devices, such as artificial joints. The material of which the joint is constructed changes completely, from cartilage and bone and ligaments to a metal or ceramic. Likewise, the structure is drastically changed, so that the blueprints for the native joint and the artificial joint look quite different from each other. And yet the joints may function quite similarly, enabling a knee that formerly could barely move to regain a virtually full range of motion.

Function refers to the operation of a molecule, a cell, a tissue, an organ, or an organ system, and activity refers to the operation of the whole organism. Consider the example of sickle cell anemia. The structural abnormality is a base-pair substitution in a portion of the gene that codes for the hemoglobin molecule. This translates into a defect in the structure of the protein, which causes it to assume an abnormal sickle shape and to become lodged in capillaries through which it should pass easily. This is a functional defect. The tendency of patients with sickle cell hemoglobin to develop anemia and sequestration crises creates limitations that interfere with daily activities, and abnormality at the level of activity. Patients with sickle cell anemia are unable to win foot races, and may not even be able to get out of bed comfortably on some days.

It is vital that future physicians understand the linkages between structure and function, and between function and activity. If we simply treat the structure, we will miss important functional implications, and if we simply treat function, we will miss important implications for what the patient is able to do. To appreciate the full implications for activity, we need to understand who patients are and what they do. Pain that one patient can easily endure may prove overwhelming to another, depending on what is going on in their lives at the time. To one patient, the ability to swing a golf club may be a crucial feature of a full life, whereas another might value especially highly the ability to sing. Because of this, the same surgical procedures might be tolerable to one and intolerable to the other. We need to ask certain questions. What does the patient care most about in life? How will different diagnostic and therapeutic options differ depending on this particular patient's point of view? We really understand the disease only insofar as we know what it means to the patient.

Participation involves the social dimension of illness. What does a letter or phone call bearing news about an abnormal diagnostic test mean to a patient? For example, suppose a patient receives a message that her screening mammogram showed an abnormality that requires further workup. What does that message mean to her? It may produce so much anxiety that she cannot sleep well or carry out her daily activities at her usual level of performance. It may upset not only the patient but her friends and family, as well. It is vital that physicians understand the human implications of such interactions, and tailor not only our bedside manner but our practice patterns in such a way that we spare patients unnecessary suffering and do what we can to promote the psychological and social well-being of patients. How can we do a better job of delivering bad news? How can we better prepare patients and families for the trials and tribulations of major surgery or anticancer chemotherapy?

When patients are told that they have cancer, they are not thinking primarily in terms of the abnormal structure of some of their cells, or the fact that a nonfunctional mass of cells is proliferating out of control and threatening their normal tissues. They think primarily in terms of what it means for their careers, their families, and their very lives. They begin to think about what it will be like to tell their spouse, their children, and their friends. They think about whether their affairs are in order. They think about all the horrible stories they have heard about the therapy for cancer, and the experiences of people they know who died of cancer. The diagnosis may incite fears of impairment and disfigurement. To young medical students, the loss of a breast or a testicle may not seem so terrible, but perhaps this is because they do not really believe it could happen to them. The more we can help learners understand the threat of illness and what it is like to cope day to day with it, the better we prepare them to care for patients in an effective and compassionate matter.

We also need to understand the social dimension of healthcare, so that we appreciate the complex relationships between different healthcare providers. How do the contributions of the family physician, pathologist, the oncologist, the surgeon, the radiologist, the dietician, the occupational therapist, the nurses, the technologists, and a host of other workers fit together to provide good care to a patient, the kind of care we would want for our spouse or sibling? Each of us needs to know what the other does, what the other needs, and what the other can offer. The more effectively we can help each of our colleagues to do their jobs, the more integrated and beneficial will be the care we provide. We need to understand not only our own specialty but the entire profession of medicine and the field of healthcare in a comprehensive fashion. If our view is fragmentary or overly simplistic, everyone suffers. On the other hand, if we can see health and disease from a truly comprehensive, multitiered perspective, both we and our patients stand to gain much.

3

Understanding Learners

Of all the men we meet with, nine parts of ten are what they are, good or evil, useful or not, by virtue of their education.

John Locke, *Some Thoughts Concerning Education*

Excelling as a Learner

If learners are to perform at their best and become the best physicians they are capable of being, it is important that we help them develop a clear vision of excellence in learning. Whether they be medical students, residents, fellows, or even practicing physicians participating in continuing medical education programs, we need to help them to see their target clearly if they are to hit it. In the case of medical students and residents, it is vital that no one regard their tenure in the training program as a period of indentured servitude, something that must be merely endured. Instead, learners gain more when they see their program as a learning opportunity designed to help them excel as learners.

The transition from medical school to residency can be particularly challenging in this regard. Throughout college and medical school, learners receive fairly clear performance expectations. They know that they want to earn high marks, and they know what level of performance is necessary to achieve them. Moreover, evaluations tend to be relatively frequent, because exams take place on a regular basis, and the results of tests are provided in relatively unequivocal terms: students' examinations are often scored numerically, and they receive grades of A, B, C, and so on. By tracking their performance over time, learners can determine whether they are doing a good job, and where necessary, take steps to improve their performance.

By contrast with premedical and medical education, many residency programs provide less clearly defined performance evaluations on a less frequent basis. Residents may meet with their program director only several times per year, and the evaluations available may be relatively vague and offer little in the way of constructive suggestions for improvement. They may include comments such as, "Great attitude," or, "Needs to read more," which can be difficult to put into practice. Moreover, we should set our sights higher than mere competence. Competence is great, but excellence is an even worthier goal, and we should attempt to develop

R.B. Gunderman, *Achieving Excellence in Medical Education*,
DOI: 10.1007/978-0-85729-307-7_3, © Springer-Verlag London Limited 2011

and articulate as clearly as possible a vision of excellent resident performance. Even if our loftiest aspirations are not achieved, their constant presence helps us perform at a higher level than we otherwise would.

To begin with, we need to dispel the enervating notion that the residents' primary goal is to survive their period of training, avoid catastrophic on-call mistakes, and prepare to pass their board examinations. Like passing a driver's test, achieving such minimal standards of performance is necessary to getting out on the road, but they do not prepare learners to flourish. Instead, they foster a lowest common denominator of performance, a desire to be merely good enough. If our learners are to thrive and achieve their full potential, we need to show them that they are capable of much more. They should aim to excel in the essential medical functions of diagnosis, consultation, and patient care, and to become the best physicians they are capable of being.

We spend thousands of hours teaching future physicians the knowledge and skills they will need to practice medicine. How many hours do we devote to developing our vision of medical excellence? This vision need not necessarily be articulated in writing, but it needs to be a frequent topic of conversation and reflection. How often do we highlight real-life examples of excellence in medicine, and how often do we take the time to discuss the sense of calling in medicine that underlies it? The goal is not so much to tell residents what their goal should be, but to encourage them to develop their own vision of medical excellence, and to evaluate their day-to-day performance in light of it. That being said, however, we should have our own vision in mind, and part of our work as educators should be sharing it with those we teach. Who are the best physicians we know, and what makes them so good? What about them would we most like to emulate, and what could we do to be more like them?

What follows is an outline of some of the general features that seem to characterize excellence among medical residents. What makes a really good resident, and what could we do to help other residents elevate their level of performance? Undoubtedly, the list of characteristics would vary somewhat from educator to educator, and some might wish to add or subtract an item or two here or there, but this discussion can at least serve as a useful point of departure for this kind of conversation.

One obvious characteristic of excellent residents is a great fund of knowledge. In any training program in any specialty, the really great residents tend to know more than their colleagues. In part, they may have devoted more time and effort to reading textbooks and journals. They may also pay more attention at teaching rounds and formal lectures. Yet the difference is not merely that they have more facts in their head. The key difference is that they are more adept at applying what they know in daily practice. When they attend a lecture, read a journal article, or discuss a case with a colleague, they are able to see how to apply that knowledge to patient care. They are able to contextualize new knowledge in such a way that it informs what they do. And it is not that they were born knowing more than everyone else. Instead, they manage to find and even create the most learning opportunities every day.

One misperception that may hamper many residents is the unrealistic view that they are supposed to know everything. If we expect ourselves to be perfect and tolerate only flawless performance, every day will be a devastating disappointment. Where knowledge is concerned, we should set high standards, but recognize that no one—not even the greatest physician who ever lived—knew everything. It is true that most great residents know more than their peers, but what really sets them apart is the importance of what they know and what they seek to learn. They are able to recognize what knowledge is more important, and to focus more of their attention on it. To some degree, standardized tests serve as a useful gauge of learning performance, but the needs of patient care, teaching, research, and service should be our ultimate guide in developing learning priorities.

Another fairly obvious characteristic of excellent residents is their skill in performing essential tasks of daily practice. Whether it be their adeptness at accessing and maintaining critical patient care information, organizing their workday, or performing a variety of diagnostic and therapeutic procedures, the best residents tend to be more skilled than their peers. Such skills are not only technical but also interpersonal. They are good at talking with patients and colleagues, and can be relied upon to convey information clearly and to do a good job of finding out what needs to be known. This is not to say, however, that they were born with such gifts. Their native manual dexterity is not necessarily superior to others'. They do, however, manifest a strong motivation to become their best, and this shows through over time in the great progress they are able to make. Despite the great importance of both, a resident's fund of knowledge and technical and interpersonal skills, other less frequently recognized characteristics tend to be equally important. The person who is chosen as chief resident is not always the one who knows the most or who displays the best performance at a particular skill. We are all familiar with residents who know more than their colleagues or who display the greatest manual dexterity, yet would never be chosen by their peers or faculty for a leadership position. If we are wise, we do not choose chief residents based strictly on their standardized test scores. Conversely, we know residents whose test scores were not the highest, yet whose overall performance would clearly win them the title of most valuable resident.

What additional characteristics do such residents possess? One such characteristic is clearly curiosity. The best residents are genuinely curious about their patients and the practice of medicine, and they treat every day as a valuable learning opportunity. The best residents may not have known more than everyone else on the first day, but they manage to wring more new insights from their work than others. Simply put, they love to learn. This love of learning manifests itself not only in their reading, but in the questions they put to patients, colleagues, and faculty. And when they learn, they are not merely collecting and cataloging facts, by seeking to understand the "How?" and "Why?" of new knowledge.

It is important that faculty members not respond to this inquisitiveness defensively. A resident who asks a lot of good questions may take more of a faculty member's time and even reveal more of the holes in the faculty member's understanding, but this deeper level of understanding will pay big dividends in terms of what excellent residents can contribute. To work with residents who really care about learning can be one of the most rewarding experiences of a medical educator, in part because it stimulates even the most accomplished among us to continue to learn and grow.

Another characteristic of great residents is their approach to errors. In the past, some programs treated errors as embarrassments that should be kept hidden, because the consequences of having an error brought to light are so dire. People whose errors were found out were either humiliated, reprimanded, or disciplined in such a way that no one wanted anyone else to know they had made a mistake. In such a culture, residents learn not to discuss or even admit their mistakes, and as a result, important opportunities to learn are lost. In an optimal learning environment, we would recognize that errors provide important learning opportunities, and seek to handle error in such a way that everyone can benefit from one another's mistakes.

It is misleading to suppose that the best residents are perfect and never make mistakes. Everyone makes mistakes. The difference between excellent residents and their peers is that the best residents make the most of their own mistakes and those of others, and put their lessons to use in improving their own approach to practice. Such mistakes range from medication errors to failure to follow up on diagnostic testing to allowing frustration or anger to interfere with professional interactions and patient care. When an error occurs, the best residents ask questions. Why did this happen? What can we learn from this mistake about our current practices? What can we do to prevent this sort of error from recurring in the future? Does this point to any broader changes we should make in the way we train residents?

Another characteristic of excellent residents is conscientiousness. Conscientiousness means more than merely working hard. It means responding to work in a certain way. Some residents attempt to get their work done as quickly as possible, with the least expenditure of effort. In some cases, this may even lead to cutting corners. This approach tends to promote preventable errors, such as failures to detect abnormalities on physical exams or to plan appropriately for patient discharge from the hospital. Other residents work very hard, but do so inefficiently, so that they work extra hours and are prone to exhausting themselves. They may be so obsessive about checking and rechecking everything that they cannot handle as much responsibility as their peers. Some residents, in other words, may prefer to do as little work as possible, and others may have difficulty discerning the appropriate amount of effort to devote to a particular objective.

Between these two extremes is a happy medium, a resident who is both effective and efficient in the use of time and who sincerely enjoys doing a good job for patients and colleagues. When we sincerely enjoy doing a good job, we are more inclined to immerse ourselves in the work for its own sake, not merely because we are afraid of getting into trouble. Those who do not enjoy the work of patient care may feel that they are merely punching a clock, working for the weekend, and this attitude shines through in the quality of their work. By contrast, those who cannot recognize when enough is enough do not really understand what they are working on, and so cannot feel comfortable that they have accomplished their mission and can move on. The best form of conscientiousness is not the result of flogging by the superego. It flows from sincere joy and pride in the work we do.

The best residents also demonstrate a high degree of personal initiative. They are not merely trying to avoid making mistakes. They are looking for opportunities to make their service run more smoothly. If they see an opportunity to contribute in some way, they seize it. If there is work to be done, they tend to volunteer to do it, in part because they enjoy helping their team to achieve its mission, and in part because they see new challenges as important learning opportunities. If there is something they need to be doing, they are less likely than others to need to be told to do it. When they are asked to do something, they set about getting it done with gusto.

Taking initiative means more than merely delivering on a job description. Great residents do what they are required to do and do it well, but are on the lookout to do more. For example, if they see a great case, they are likely to write it up for presentation or publication. If they realize that the curriculum on a particular rotation could be improved, they take the initiative to suggest changes, and to help bring those changes about. Left to their own devices, they tend to improve the programs of which they are a part. They see the program not merely as a springboard to their own success, but as an organization to whose mission they are committed, and to which they can make an important contribution.

Another related characteristic of excellent residents is reliability. When someone asks a great resident to tend to something, they can be relied upon to see that it gets done. This reliability manifests itself in both obvious and not so obvious ways. In obvious terms, it means that great residents show up for work on time, stay till the work gets done, and can be counted on to be where they are supposed to be. In less obvious terms, this reliability shines through in the everyday tasks of medical practice. The best residents obtain their own histories, make sure that all the laboratory results are checked every day, follow up with patients, never cut corners in collecting or analyzing data, and prepare thoroughly for new challenges. Not only faculty but fellow residents, medical students, and other allied health personnel have confidence in reliable residents.

Great residents are also generally affable people. They need not be the most popular people in their programs or the life of the party at social functions. They need not be the best looking or best dressed. They do, however, tend to be well liked by almost everyone, because they treat people fairly and respectfully, and manifest a genuine interest in their well being. Such residents talk with others, and know what is going on in others' lives. They know who is getting engaged to be married, or who has a baby on the way. They also know who is having difficulties, and do what they can to help. Above all, they treat everyone they work with as human beings. They do not have one standard of conduct for their superiors and another standard for those below them on the ladder of authority.

A characteristic of many, though not all excellent, residents is their range of interests and responsibilities outside medicine. Many have unusual life experiences, wider professional backgrounds, or special extracurricular interests. Some bring past work experience in such areas as entrepreneurship, teaching, or information technology, which enriches their medical work. Others bring a certain intellectual maturity and balance to their work because of outside avocations, such as dance, woodworking, religious service, or coaching a youth athletic team or leading a scout troop. Family life, especially marriage and parenthood, may contribute to professional maturity, as well. Having children of their own enables some residents to view day-to-day challenges from a somewhat larger perspective that makes difficulties seem a bit less overwhelming.

Above all, excellent residents manifest admirable character. They are honest, unselfish, and genuinely understanding of others. In an important sociological study of residency training, Charles Bosk identified two types of resident errors: technical and normative. Technical errors, such as missing a physical examination finding or failing to prescribe the appropriate medication, are generally forgiven, as long as the resident makes an effort to learn from them. Normative errors, by contrast, include lack of dedication and frank dishonesty. These sorts of errors are not easily forgiven, because they indicate a deficiency not only of knowledge or skill, but of character. Great residents are, above all, people we can trust to do what is right.

In sum, it is by helping faculty and, especially, residents develop a clearer and more complete vision of excellence in residency that we can best prepare residents to excel. This is our target, and only by clearly seeing our target are we prepared to hit it. Once we define such a vision, we can use it to guide our growth and development not only during residency but throughout our careers, because the characteristics of great residents are also the characteristics of great physicians.

Learners' Views of Excellence

Most of us would like to excel at what we do, but few of us have devoted much time and energy to the study of excellence. Similarly, we want to avoid failure, but most of us do not learn as much as we could from our disappointments. Often we are too relieved or even exulted in our successes to step back and think through what we did right, and the pain of failure may be so great that we simply want to put it behind us as soon as possible. Yet, if our learners are going to improve their performance, it is important that we foster reflection on the question of why, despite equal levels of intelligence and experience, some people perform at a high level and other people perform relatively poorly.

A wealth of educational research indicates that our very ideas of what constitutes success and failure differ widely, and that these differing understandings powerfully influence our level of achievement. In what respects do high achievers differ from low achievers? Some of the most important distinguishing features have been elucidated by a group of psychologists developing what has come to be called attribution theory. There are some learner attitudes and perceptions we cannot change, but there are others that we can revise, and doing so can help learners such as medical students, residents, and practicing physicians perform at a higher level.

The factors that either enhance or detract from high performance can be divided into two categories, extrinsic and intrinsic. Extrinsic factors concern decisions made by people other than learners themselves, such as faculty members. These include expectations, reactions of praise or blame, and rewards or punishments. Do we expect learners to perform well or poorly? Do we offer frequent praise when learners perform well, or do we simply withhold blame? Do we lead primarily with a carrot or with a stick? Intrinsic factors pertain to learners themselves, and include their expectations, their level of motivation to perform at their best, and the level of challenge they experience in learning. We tend to feel relatively little sense of accomplishment if our learning tasks do not challenge us in any meaningful way. By contrast, a high sense of achievement may flow from a moderately difficult task, one that demands our full concentration and effort. If learners are to perform at their best, it is important that they approach learning tasks with at least a moderately high level of intrinsic engagement and a reasonably high expectation of success. If they see no importance to what they are learning, or if they think they have little chance of success in learning it, they are unlikely to perform at their best.

Thus we need to challenge learners but not overwhelm them. If they feel they never had a chance or did not need to make an effort, the learning experience is likely to provide little benefit. In educating medical students, for example, we need to ensure that we tailor learning tasks to their particular level. What can a second-year medical student be expected to know, and how does it differ from what a fourth-year student knows? If we pay close attention to learners, the same clinical case that helps to reinforce important anatomical and physiological principles for a second-year student can also help a fourth-year student consolidate important diagnostic and therapeutic principles. This can only work, however, if we know the learners, and operate with appropriate expectations.

Learning environments can powerfully influence learners' expectations for themselves, as well as how they appraise their own performance. If we are confronted with learning tasks for which we lack the means to prepare, we are less likely to feel proud of the work we have done, even if we happen to succeed. Our probability of success declines when we lack preparation, and confronting learners with questions they cannot know the answer to can leave them feeling discouraged and undermine their motivation to learn. We can apply this principle in teaching by structuring learning experiences in such a way that learners can easily see the relevance of what they already know to the learning task at hand.

We can, for example, help medical students and residents become more effective clinical consultants by presenting them with situations where they are asked to interact with colleagues in formulating diagnostic and therapeutic plans for patients. From the first days of medical school, students can be asked to think in terms of what they would recommend for a particular patient. In the beginning, questions can focus more on what additional information they need and how they would go about acquiring it, and as they progress, they can be asked to use what they know to choose between different available options for diagnostic testing and the like. In this manner, students do not feel so unprepared when they begin to care for real patients.

We can further enhance learner effectiveness by making clear the level of effort we expect. The goal is to provide learners a sense that they enjoy substantial control over their own educational destiny. Do we provide medical students and residents realistic sets of learning objectives, and do we tailor daily teaching and assessment to them? It is no use setting expectations so low that no one could ever fail. But they do need to be explicit enough that learners are able to discern not only what they should be studying but also what they should be able to do with what they are learning. A good example is the way we teach cardiopulmonary resuscitation, where we not only expect learners to pass a written exam, but also to actually perform each of the maneuvers.

If we want to perform better, we need to develop a sense that we can make things happen, as opposed to the sense that things merely happen to us. The key is the locus of control. Learners who see the locus of control as lying outside themselves are much less likely to see a strong connection between the choices they make and their level of performance. When things do not go as expected, they blame it on forces over which they have no control, such as bad luck or the failures of others. By contrast, learners who exhibit a high sense of personal efficacy are likely to regard setbacks not as the work of some inscrutable, and malign outside force, but as their own mistakes from which they can learn and improve in the future. Such learners study their experiences, both failures and successes, to determine what they could do differently. They recognize that they are not in complete control, but they seek out those aspects that they can influence and try to influence them more positively in the future.

One means of fostering this kind of self-awareness among learners is the so-called critical incident approach. How does it work? At the conclusion of a learning task, learners are asked to reflect on their performance and to determine why they performed as they did. If our organizations are to perform at their best, we need to attract people who are accustomed to reflecting on and learning from their experiences. If we ask a candidate to tell the story of one of their greatest successes or failures and they cannot think of one, that is a bad sign. The same is true if they have no idea why things turned out as they did, or if they keep attributing the result to external forces. We want learners to see themselves not as victims, but as cocreators of their own level of excellence.

To foster this kind of self-awareness, we need to encourage learners to step back and reflect on their performance, and to develop the habit of doing so on a regular basis. How often do we sit down with medical students or residents and ask them to tell the story of one of their biggest successes or failures? Why did it turn out that way? What could they do differently in the future to improve the result? If learners do not spend at least part of their time reflecting on their own performance, looking into the mirror, so to speak, they will be less well equipped to learn from their practice and continue to improve in the future.

It is not enough, however, merely to regard the locus of control as internal. It is equally important whether we see the internal factors as fixed or alterable. An internal factor that many of us tend to regard as fixed is innate ability. It is sad but true that many young people develop low expectations of themselves as a result of just a few disappointments. For example, students suppose that they just cannot do math, or they lack the manual dexterity necessary to become a surgeon. In short, they develop a "can't do" attitude, supposing that they must have been absent on the day a particular ability was distributed. Learners who interpret their poor performance in terms of their own intrinsic lack of ability are much less likely than others to feel challenged by disappointments or to make efforts to change their approach in the future. Instead, they are likely simply to give up. This is not to say that each of us does not have limitations. However, we should not be so quick to invoke our limitations as the explanation for our disappointing performances.

We need to encourage learners to shift their focus from ability to effort. When we fail, we can either say, "I am just not good at this," or we can say, "I wonder what I could have done differently." If the goal is to foster the attitude that obstacles can be overcome and to improve, then we need to foster the latter perspective. The question is not, "What am I capable of?" but, "How can I make an even stronger effort?" Do we as educators regard students' performance primarily as an indicator of how smart they are, or as an indicator of their level of effort? Insofar as possible, we should attempt to think in terms of effort, because our attitudes may powerfully influence how learners come to think themselves. What is our attitude toward mistakes? Do we see every error as a sign that we are failures, or do we see it as a learning opportunity? People who never make mistakes have ceased to learn, and unless we can claim to know everything, none of us can afford to stop learning. Every error can be a steppingstone to excellence, by helping us better discern what works. By contrast, labeling ourselves as failures just makes us even less likely to perform well in the future. Learners who believe they lack ability, that the challenges before them are simply too difficult, or that they have no control over their own destiny are much more likely to consider themselves failures than people who interpret setbacks as learning opportunities.

As Thomas Edison repeatedly emphasized, perseverance is a more constant feature of high achievers than genius. Medical students and residents are accustomed to thinking of themselves as bright people, and expect to succeed. In some cases, a disappointing performance may leave them at a loss. When that happens we cannot afford to act mules, who merely keep trying the same thing over and over again, only harder. Insanity was once defined as the expectation of deriving different results from doing the same thing. In contrast to the mule, when the fox fails, he changes his approach and does something different. Effort is not merely bull-headedness, but the wealth of experience and ingenuity that lies at our disposal.

Many features of medical education tend to discourage this attitude. For example, our written examinations generally emphasize conformity. There is one right answer, and it is the same right answer for every learner. We reward memorization and recall. Not only does this discourage the attitudes of skepticism and creativity on which the future of medicine depend, but it also tends to undermine learners' capacity to respond effectively to setbacks. Winston Churchill performed poorly in subjects such as mathematics, and graduated near the bottom of his class in secondary

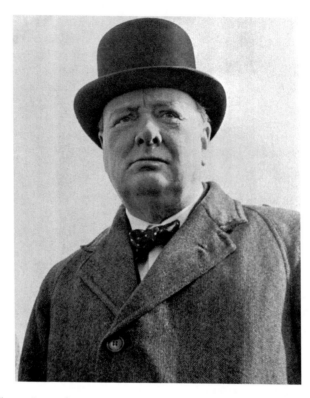

Fig.3.1 Sir Winston Leonard Spencer-Churchill (1874–1965). Despite a speech impediment and a scholastic record so poor that his father despaired over his future, Churchill went on to serve twice as British prime minister, lead his nation during the darkest hours of the Second World War, win the Nobel Prize in Literature, and become the first person ever recognized as an honorary citizen of the USA. In a speech at Dundee, Scotland in 1908, he asked, "What is the use of living, if it be not to strive for noble causes and to make this muddled world a better place for those who will live in it after we are gone?" (Courtesy of Wikimedia Commons)

school (Fig. 3.1). He always knew, however, that he had a greater destiny in life, and despite his parents' and teachers' despair, he kept doing what seemed important to him. Eventually, his efforts paid off, and he became one of the most important political leaders of the twentieth century and won a Nobel Prize in literature.

Churchill's story reminds us of the importance of risk taking. Victory alone is not what is most important. What is most important is performing at our best, and making the best contribution we can. If we restrict ourselves to challenges we can easily overcome, we are unlikely to improve. By contrast, if we want to become our best, we need to choose meaningful challenges, to take risks, and to accept the possibility of failure and defeat. Playing it safe is a recipe for indolence and mediocrity. The best leaders are those who encourage not only themselves but those around them to strive beyond what we are certain we are capable of.

What risks could medical students take? Here are some ideas. Find a question in medicine to which no one knows the answer and develop a plan to answer it.

Develop a lesson to teach colleagues about a key concept in medicine. Take a course in a nonmedical subject, such as history, philosophy, or art. Draft a one- to two-page critique of a class you are taking with suggestions for improvement, and share it with the instructor. Write brief biographical sketches of a dozen of your colleagues. Spend a month helping to deliver healthcare in a foreign country. Such experiences are important not merely in their own right but because they encourage learners to begin to think in broader terms about the challenges open to them.

If we are going to perform at our best, we need to clearly understand what we are trying to do. If our aim is merely to avoid mistakes, we are selling short both ourselves and our profession. The best learners are those who seek out challenges and continue to question and grow throughout their careers. We need to look beyond the content of our textbooks and consider the effects of our educational programs on learners' habits and self-perceptions. All of us are capable of more than we think, and if we recognize what is necessary to unlock more of that potential, we can perform at a higher level of excellence.

Attracting Medical Students to Understaffed Fields

A shortage of physicians in any medical specialty or subspecialty represents a threat not only to patients but to the field of medicine. When the supply of physicians in any field is insufficient to meet the demand for their services, patient care ideally provided by specialists is likely to be provided by nonspecialists, or perhaps even by nonphysicians. A workforce shortage also interferes with the ability of physicians in understaffed specialties to develop good working liaisons with physicians in other fields. This may compromise patient care by interfering with the development of effective interdisciplinary collaborations. Finally, a workforce shortage may make the field even less attractive to medical students who might otherwise enter it, because they see practitioners as overworked and stressed out.

The etiologies of workforce shortages are complex. For example, production may be insufficient. Consider the advice given to students during their training. During the early and mid-1990s, students at many US medical schools were discouraged from entering subspecialties, which were seen as oversupplied, and encouraged to enter primary care fields. By the mid to late 1990s, the number of applicants to specialties such as anesthesiology and radiology had fallen markedly. Other factors affect demand. These include population growth (which stimulates demand for all medical specialties), demographics (the demand for geriatricians increases with the number of elderly people), and the introduction of additional services by specialists in the field (such as the effect of the introduction of MRI on the demand for radiologists).

If we are to cope effectively with workforce shortages, we need to gain a clearer understanding of the factors that influence medical students' career decision making. We need to understand what factors weigh most heavily in their career choices. What makes one medical specialty more attractive than another? Why do some medical specialties seem so unattractive to so many students? In this sphere, perception is more important than reality. How do medical students appraise the strengths of an understaffed field? What do they see as its weaknesses? What features do they find attractive, and which tend to drive them away?

One factor that may undermine student interest is income. Students may be attracted to relatively highly remunerated specialties, and less attracted to fields that pay relatively poorly. Some may fear that a field is too sub specialized, narrowing their focus to an excessive degree to only a particular organ system and thus drawing them away from the "whole" patient. Others may worry that a specialty is too broad, rendering them "jacks of all trades but masters of none." Some may fear that opting for an understaffed medical specialty would leave them little time or energy to pursue a life outside medicine. Similarly, they may worry that faculty members in the field are too thinly stretched to provide good training. Some medical students may also have doubts about the patient populations characteristically served by the field. Some may find working with sick children emotionally stressful, and others may find a career caring for elderly patients with chronic diseases too depressing.

If we are to address the perceptual factors that contribute to workforce shortages in medicine, we need to get inside the minds of students to understand how they see each specialty. If we gain a clear understanding of those forces, we will be in a much stronger position to develop effective responses. The specific factors will vary from specialty to specialty, but there are also some general factors from which most specialty could benefit.

Broadly speaking, there are two fundamentally different types of factors that affect student interest in a specialty, with two corresponding strategies for enhancement. These are extrinsic factors and intrinsic factors. Intrinsic factors concern the nature of the work performed by physicians in the specialty. Extrinsic factors lie outside the work itself. These might include compensation, flexibility of scheduling, ease of entry into the field, availability of allied health personnel in support roles, and the availability of new technologies to increase efficiency and decrease the less engaging aspects of clinical practice. Although such extrinsic factors certainly deserve to be addressed, they are not the focus of this discussion. What follows are brief descriptions of a number of the intrinsic factors, as well as strategies for addressing them.

One such factor is confidence. When medical students are exposed to a particular medical specialty during their training, do they develop sufficient confidence in their abilities to begin feeling comfortable at applying such knowledge and skills to the care of patients? In an effort to impress students with how smart we are or demanding our field is, how often do we simply overwhelm students with information, leaving them with the feeling that they could never approach mastery? One effective response to this problem would be to develop a clearly defined curriculum of what students could reasonably be expected to master and then giving them an opportunity to apply that knowledge during their training experience in the field. What specifically are they expected to learn and to be able to do, and what opportunities will they enjoy to contribute to the care of patients? The goal is not to make things unrealistically easy for students, but to give them an opportunity to develop a graduated mastery, or at least competency. No one, not even the most accomplished expert in the field, knows everything, and we can do our field a favor by giving students an opportunity to feel they have acquitted themselves well as learners.

A related factor is expertise. Although similar at first glance to confidence, expertise involves a different dimension of mastery, namely, depth of understanding. If expectations for students are set at the right level, they can achieve most mastery and confidence in those learning objectives. They cannot, however, become masters in the field, because there simply is no time. True expertise would require years, perhaps even decades. They can, however, get a taste of expertise by choosing a particular question or topic in the field and exploring it in depth, and then making a presentation on it at the end of their training experience. For example, a student might choose to investigate a particular disease, test, patient, or clinical presentation. One way of making learning especially rewarding to students is to seek out opportunities to put their new-found expertise to use in the care of patients. For example, if a student has made a particular inpatient her focus of study, she can be called upon to provide information needed for discharge planning and the like. There is a special kind of satisfaction to be found from knowing one thing really well, and we should make an effort to allow students to experience it.

Another factor is the academic side of the field. Student interest in a field may be enhanced by giving them an opportunity to participate in such academic pursuits as education and research. Every student can learn enough about a subject to teach it well to someone else, whether a patient, a more junior student, or a health professional in another field. Likewise, every medical student is intelligent enough to contribute in some way to investigation. The key is to move students out of the role of passive recipients of knowledge and into the active role of sharing or advancing it. The very brightest of our students will not be fully engaged by merely memorizing what someone else tells them they need to know. What they need are opportunities to see what they are capable of and to spread their intellectual wings.

Another factor that can influence student interest in a field is teaching excellence. We need to ensure that we as faculty members care about education out of more than a sense that our jobs may be on the line if we do not do at least a passable job of teaching. Of course, education should be a meaningful factor in career advancement, including promotion and tenure. Yet the best teaching is grounded in something more: a sense that education is one of the highest callings of a physician, and that excelling as an educator is one of the most rewarding aspects of a career in medicine. How can we help faculty find more fulfillment as educators? One way is to help them perform better at it. There is no question that some people seem to be more naturally gifted as teachers than others, but teaching is also a learnable art, and given the right opportunities, all of us can improve. Our career choices are powerfully influenced by the teachers with whom we come in contact, and specialties that boast the best teachers in the medical school will enjoy a competitive advantage in recruiting medical students. We can encourage good teaching by developing and supporting faculty development programs, and by recognizing outstanding teachers appropriately.

A related factor concerns the opportunities faculty members enjoy to teach. If the clinical workday is so overstuffed with patient care responsibilities that there is no time to seize important teaching opportunities, then education will suffer. This is not to say that academic physicians cannot be busy, but only that we cannot be too busy. We need sufficient time for meaningful educational interaction with students, including, above all, time at the point of patient care. Formal lectures and other didactic learning opportunities are also important, and must be protected if the education is to thrive. To find such time, it may be necessary for departments to add to their support staff, to install new technology to increase clinical efficiency, or even to permit an expanded workday to permit more time for student learning. The amount of time involved need not be great. Just one 30-min session each day, or only a few days per week, can make a big difference in terms of student perception of a field's educational commitment.

Another often unrecognized factor is the presence of role models. Do students feel that the faculties in the field are good mentors? Do they see in them their future selves? Do they feel welcome and appreciated for their efforts? Do they feel that they can approach faculty members for advice? Above all, do they admire them? It is important that students see in faculty members a sincere dedication to the best interests of patients, and the fulfillment that grows out of it. We cannot afford to neglect the role of inspiration in career choice.

Finally, we need to ensure that medical students enjoy meaningful opportunities to contribute to the care of patients. Many young people enter medical school in the hope of making a difference in the lives of others, and it is primarily through face-to-face contact with patients that such satisfaction is likely to emerge. This is the very motivation that medicine most needs to reward. Hence, we need to design the training experience accordingly, so that medical students can experience what it feels like to have a patient call you "my doctor." Likewise, medical students should enjoy meaningful responsibility for interacting with other health professionals in the care of their patients, including writing chart notes, requesting tests and procedures, and representing their patients in case conferences.

Learning to Care for Ourselves

"Old Doc Rivers," a short story by the physician-poet William Carlos Williams, beautifully portrays the tension between an early twentieth century physician's dedication to patients and his inability to recognize and respond to his own health-related impairments (Fig. 3.2). On the plus side, Doc Rivers would "go anywhere, anytime, for anybody," and his flashes of brilliance as a diagnostician and therapist establish his reputation as a local legend. Yet his punishing schedule exacts an immense toll, his reliability progressively declines, and he ends up ruined by alcohol and drugs. Through this beautiful story, Williams confronts physicians with two vital questions: how can we strike the appropriate balance between caring for patients and caring for self, and what can we do to help future physicians find their own appropriate balance point?

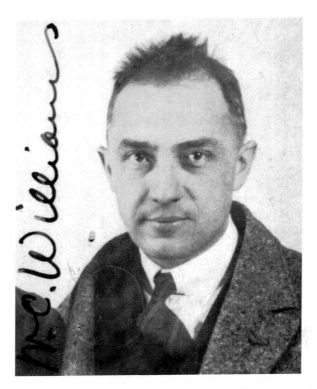

Fig. 3.2 William Carlos Williams (1883–1963). Physician-poet Williams practiced medicine in Rutherford, New Jersey, where he was reputed to have delivered more than 3,000 babies. In his autobiography, Williams wrote of the relationship between words and illness. While medical educators sometimes treat the patient's words as mere means to arriving at a diagnosis, Williams argued that illnesses are in fact vehicles for bringing us face-to-face with human beings: "We begin to see that the underlying meaning of all they want to tell us and have always failed to communicate is the poem, the poem which their lives are being lived to realize. No one will believe it. And it is the actual words, as we hear them spoken under all circumstances, which contain it. It is actually there, in the life before us, every minute that we are listening, a rarest element—not in our imaginations but there, there in fact. It is that essence which is hidden in the very words which are going in at our ears and from which we must recover underlying meaning as realistically as we recover metal out of ore" (Courtesy of Wikimedia Commons)

Dedication to patients is both necessary and appropriate, but not when it begins to seriously encroach on our ability to attend to our own health needs. If we fail to attend to our own health, we may undermine our fitness to practice medicine. Many disorders can interfere with the quality of a physician's work, including such diverse conditions as influenza, cancer, Parkinson's disease, and substance abuse. On the positive side, good health plays an important role in enabling us to perform at our best. A pianist produces better music with a well-maintained and properly tuned instrument, and a similar principle applies to a physician who is flourishing biologically and psychologically.

Patients, families, communities, and the profession of medicine have a legitimate interest in the health of physicians. We bear a professional responsibility to educate future physicians to recognize their health-related limitations and take appropriate steps to safeguard those who depend on them. No patient should suffer harm because a physician is too sleep deprived, febrile, intoxicated, or simply too distressed to perform at a sufficient level. Depending on circumstances, this may require rescheduling a patient's visit or arranging for a colleague to serve in our place. What might seem at first glance an admission of weakness turns out to offer powerful testimony to the strength of our dedication to patients.

Future physicians need to be prepared to assume the role of recipients, not just providers of care. To be sure, some people may prefer not to see us as vulnerable to the same injuries and ailments that beset those we care for. Yet we must guard against perpetuating the misconception that the white coat is a cloak of invulnerability. The lifetime mortality rate of physicians is no less than that of patients, and even the healthiest physicians, after curing many patients, eventually fall ill and die. By helping learners to appreciate that physicians are cut from the same cloth as our patients, we lay the groundwork for greater compassion and enable our future colleagues to put the welfare of patients above their own determination and pride.

Physicians need to appreciate the Socratic maxim, "Know yourself." Are we educating future physicians to recognize when their own health status compromises patient care, and showing them the steps they can take to ensure that patient needs are met? Equally important, are we educating them to discern the signs of impairment in colleagues, and instilling in them a willingness to intervene on patients' behalf? Medicine thrives as a profession only so long as it monitors its own ranks. Physicians have a duty to watch out for one another, and to subordinate the understandable desire to avoid embarrassment and confrontation to the good of patients.

Yet we need to exercise caution lest we forget the limits of health as a medical priority. Reasonable patients would never choose a physician based solely on his or her health status. We cannot infer a high degree of medical knowledge, skill, or dedication from a slim waistline, a low blood pressure, or an ideal serum lipid profile. In fact, an excessive preoccupation with personal health may prevent us from devoting sufficient time and attention to the needs of patients. From the patient's point of view, there is comfort in knowing that a physician is prepared to skip occasional meals or sacrifice a few hours' sleep to provide care.

Health is limited in a further sense. An educational approach that does a good job of protecting patients from physicians' impairments may not fare so well at promoting excellence in medicine. Like a driver education program that focuses on preventing traffic infractions, it may draw too much attention away from ultimately more important questions: What, professionally speaking, is our destination? How, in terms of our day-to-day commitments, are we getting there? How personally fulfilling is the journey? Every driver wants to avoid getting a traffic ticket or injuring others, but there is more to a successful journey than safety. Physicians would never select as their epitaph, "He took great care of himself," or "She scrupulously avoided impairment."

Future physicians need to feel the force of this statement: the most worthy aim of a life in medicine is not to satisfy minimal standards of safety and competence, but to excel as a physician. Focusing too much attention on impairment and its remediation may distract us from what is required for us to perform at our best. We need to attend to physician health in a way that situates the prevention, diagnosis, and treatment of physician impairment as a byproduct of a higher pursuit. The best protection against impairment is not a rigorous system of detection and enforcement, but an approach to the practice of medicine that promotes genuine fulfillment, enabling physicians to do to the best of their abilities the very things that are most worth doing.

Future physicians will do better work if they have good work to do. Such work is characterized much less by extrinsic rewards such as power, fame, or money than by the intrinsic rewards of the work itself. Are we helping learners to grow and develop through their labors? Are we teaching them to practice medicine in a way that accords with their highest aspirations, the ideals that drew them to a career in medicine in the first place and have animated this venerable profession throughout its history? And most importantly, are we providing them the opportunity to make a significant difference in the lives of the patients, families, and communities they serve? If the answer is yes, then impairment is less likely to become an issue.

Medical students, residents, and practicing physicians who derive genuine fulfillment from the pursuit of medicine's highest aspirations are less likely to become discouraged, suffer burn out, and neglect themselves. Far from finding their work a burden, they tend to cherish it as a privilege, one of life's dearest opportunities to develop and express the best that is in them. They need not flog themselves from day to day to keep going, because they are drawing from one of the most invigorating wellsprings of inspiration available to human beings—the sense that we are achieving our full potential by enriching the lives of others. Future physicians may make a living by what they get, but they will make a life by what they give.

Some commentators have suggested that the term "healthcare system" is a misnomer. They argue that what we really have is not a healthcare system but a sickcare system, which does well at rescuing patients from medical catastrophes but performs poorly at preventing disease and promoting health. In addition, they regard the system itself as anything but systematic, a patchwork quilt of poorly aligned incentives and outcomes. The accuracy of such assessments is open to debate, but one thing seems clear. If physicians are to fulfill our mission to promote the well-being of patients and communities, we need to understand the appropriate role of health in fostering rich, full lives.

The word health derives from an Old English word that means whole. To become and remain whole, future physicians need to learn to approach health like a symphonist. Merely getting each piece in perfect working order is not enough. We need virtuoso musicians, who know how to play their parts to perfection, in ways that harmonize perfectly with the other performers. Physicians may be able to get the cells and organs in good working order, but if the body is not aligned with the mind and the soul, the result will be cacophony. Only when the lower parts harmonize with the higher can we perform well and contribute fully to the larger symphony of excellent medicine.

The greatest threat facing medicine today is not a deficit of sleep, nutrition, or longevity. Nor is it a deficiency in healthcare reimbursement or even the erosion of professional autonomy. The greatest threat facing medicine today is a deficit of inspiration, what we might call "inspiration deficit disorder." The future vitality of physicians and the wholeness of the profession itself depend above all on our ability to help learners connect deeply with the inherently inspiring aspects of medicine. If we can help position them on a trajectory toward this higher end, the lower ends, including the health of physicians, will tend to find their proper orientation.

4

Promoting Learners

The best way to understand is to do. That which we learn most thoroughly, and remember the best, is what we have in a way taught ourselves.

Immanuel Kant, *Thoughts on Education*

Focusing on Learners

Especially in medicine, most of us are familiar with educational approaches that are instructor centered. The instructor is the single most active person in the learning environment, and bears responsibility for determining what is taught, how it is taught, when it is taught, and how learner performance is assessed. Often underlying instructor-centered approaches to education is the view that learners such as medical students are basically empty receptacles waiting to be filled up with the knowledge the instructor contains.

Despite the great prevalence of instructor-centered models in medical education, a great deal of investigation and discussion in the contemporary literature favors a more learner-centered approach to education. This is grounded in the insight that the goal of education is less to exercise instructors than to cultivate knowledge and skills in learners. In other words, education is more about learners than instructors, and it is fitting that educational approaches be more tailored to the opportunities the learner presents.

Many, if not most medical educators, have little or no formal background as educators. Except by example, no one ever taught us how to teach effectively. We have all but tacitly accepted such insidious educational concepts as the fund of knowledge. Operating on this principle, we suppose that our goal is to increase our learners' fund of knowledge in a relevant subject area. Such a concept is highly instructor-centered, however, and all but inevitably promotes an instructor-centered educational approach. We find ourselves operating as though there was a knowledge level in the mind of the learner, and all we need to do to determine it is insert a dipstick. The higher the level, the more knowledge we have successfully imparted. Yet, learners' minds are more than tanks, and knowledge is more than a liquid with which we fill them. If we are to meet the needs of learners more effectively, it is vital that we develop a clearer understanding of what goes on in their minds.

R.B. Gunderman, *Achieving Excellence in Medical Education*,
DOI: 10.1007/978-0-85729-307-7_4, © Springer-Verlag London Limited 2011

Sometimes the sheer volume of information that medical students and residents face leaves them feeling oppressed or nervous. They quite reasonably deduce that they will not be able to learn everything, and seek out guidance on what they really need to know. In the most stressful situations, this boils down to the effort to discern what will be on the test. Learning comes to be directed by evaluation, and soon learners have lost their focus on what they will need to know to excel as physicians. In the ideal situation, learners are focused on the latter, on what a good physician needs to know. To foster such learning, educators can ensure that learners face problems that closely approximate those they will face in actual practice.

Here, using patients and case histories as the focus can be extremely helpful. When a patient presents with a particular problem, what sorts of information does the physician need to seek, which aspects of the history and physical examination are most appropriate, and which tests are most likely to be helpful? When medical students begin their discussion of acid–base balance with a particular patient in respiratory alkalosis or metabolic acidosis, they are able to situate the discussion in a clinically relevant context from the outset. Such problem-based approaches also put students in the role of problem solvers, not mere memorizers. The knowledge they acquire, therefore, tends to be usable, as opposed to the frequently inert form of knowledge that memorization spawns. Learners are not merely trying to recall what they were told, but to use knowledge to solve a problem similar to those they will face in medical practice.

Learner-centered education advances an attitude of respect for learners. Those who choose careers in medicine are usually very bright and capable people, and they enjoy a challenge. They are unlikely to respond to their fullest capability if they are treated like small children and simply told what to do. We should let them know that their own learning needs and preferences have shaped their educational program. They are not like passengers in a car on an amusement park ride, but like members of a team exploring a new geographical region. Their route is not entirely predetermined, and even their destination is to some degree subject to their own discretion. They are not sheets of metal moving along a conveyor belt, about to be stamped into a particular shape. At their best, they are active participants and even collaborators in their own education, and our mission as educators is to enable them to realize that potential.

If we do not respect learners' potential to function as coinvestigators and even codirectors of their own education, we may foster an attitude of "learned helplessness," where formerly bright and self-directed learners become increasingly reliant on instructors to tell them what to do. How well would such an attitude prepare them for the challenge of lifelong learning that a career in medicine represents? How will they know what books and journals to read, what continuing education courses to attend, and how well they are doing as learners? Will we keep giving them reading assignments and exams their whole lives? No. To prepare them to flourish as learners, we need to give them an active role in determining what to learn and how to go about learning it. We need not begin the class telling medical students what they should want to learn. We can begin the class by getting them talking about what they want to learn and why, and we can tailor the syllabus, at least in part, to what they say.

Learners do not arrive in medical school or residency as Descartes' blank tablets. They bring with them prior experiences and a desire to help shape their own learning. What do they know already? How might the subject matter of this particular course or clinical rotation fit more dynamically into their current understanding? Even first-year medical students have had experience with healthcare. What "cases" do they bring with them on day one? By bringing to light and making use of what learners already know, we make the relevance of the material much more transparent, because the learners themselves helped to supply much of it. Moreover, we also help learners develop as true learners, not mere memorizers, by challenging them to play an active role in shaping their own educational experience.

Understanding the questions and experiences learners bring to the table can become increasingly difficult, the greater the gap that separates instructors and learners. It is therefore especially important to get to know and understand novices. If we are not careful, we may find ourselves using terms and concepts that are unfamiliar to learners, and instruction ends up going "over their heads." It is simply a mistake to overlook the important differences that separate first-year medical students from fourth-year medical students, or fourth-year medical students from third-year residents. What works well with one group of learners may fail miserably with another, either because it assumes too much knowledge and clinical experience, or underestimates the capability of learners. What bores or insults one group may totally overwhelm another. And sometimes the relevant gradations are measured not in years but in months or, in some cases, even days.

Showing respect for learners makes them want to work harder by paying attention and striving to do well. When learners see that instructors take seriously what they already know, they will do so as well. If learners think that instructors are fiercely on the lookout for every mistake so that we can pounce on it and humiliate them, they are likely to become more and more reticent about asking questions and offering insights. On the other hand, if they sense that identifying and redressing lacunae in their understanding is regarded as an important opportunity, then they are likely to develop into more self-critical and self-directed learners. Sometimes the best response to a learner's question is not the answer, but another question. What learners do not know is not an empty chasm that we must close. Instead, it is fertile soil on which to sow the seeds of additional learning (Fig. 4.1). It is an opportunity for educators to do what we do best—to teach. More importantly, it is also an opportunity to help learners achieve one of their greatest missions, namely, to enhance their ability to learn.

When we work with learners, we want them to understand that we are not merely talking to them, but conversing with them. Our primary mission is not to make ourselves feel more important or advance our careers. We are not showing off how much we know. Rather, we are attempting to help learners learn what they most need to know. Therefore, the most important person in the classroom is not the teacher, but the student. We need to think less about our own performance and

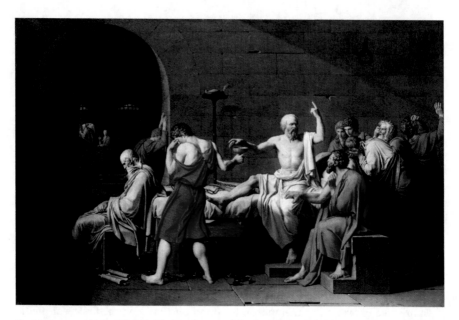

Fig. 4.1 Socrates (469–399 BC). Known as one of the founders of philosophy, Socrates is shown here in Jacques-Louis David's 1787 painting depicting his death. Having just taken the poison that will end his life, carrying out a sentence handed down by a jury of his fellow Athenians, Socrates died as he lived, pursuing wisdom and drawing his comrades' attention to higher matters. Despite his timeless status as one of the wisest human beings, Socrates repeatedly professed his own ignorance, and frequently responded to learners' questions with questions of his own. His goal, it seems, was to get us thinking for ourselves (Courtesy of Wikimedia)

more about the performance of learners. Are we challenging them in meaningful ways, not merely to stay awake or to write down everything we are saying, but to think critically and creatively, and to solve problems? When we evaluate students, we need to look beyond mere selection and sorting of students, and focus instead on evaluation as a formative opportunity. Does our evaluation fan the flames of their motivation and help them do a better job of learning? The goal is not to pass some examination, but to become a fine physician.

One thing we know about the maturation of learners is that the more mature we become, the more intrinsically motivated we tend to become. In other words, our learning becomes more and more motivated by our own needs and interests, rather than outside requirements. Grades can become a self-defeating reward system, if they keep us focused on external as opposed to internal motivations and rewards for learning. We must prepare learners for a professional career in which they will no longer receive grades at the end of every term, and when they will have to decide for themselves what to learn and whether they are doing a good job of learning it.

What motivates mature learners? To a large part it is pure curiosity, the desire to understand something for its own sake. Another important motivator is the questions that arise during daily practice. Another is the opportunity to help a patient. In these situations, people are trying to learn not because someone tells them they must, or because they want to impress someone else, but because the knowledge itself is important to them. These intrinsic motivators have at their core curiosity and the desire to excel at our craft. Are we becoming the physicians to whom colleagues will turn when they have questions?

The purpose in highlighting learner-centered education is not to suggest that we should be designing individualized and unique curricula for every learner. However, it is possible for many of us to employ a richer and more varied educational approach. Different learners learn best in different contexts and by different approaches, and we can help our learners discover what works best for them by presenting them with different possibilities and encouraging them to reflect on their learning experiences. Some do best learning alone and others in small groups. Some do best reading the material and others do best when they hear it. Electronic educational media offer additional opportunities to interact with the material in varied ways. Learners are, after all, human beings, and no two are exactly alike. If we treat them as though they were simply carbon copies of a single learner, then we will be doing both them and ourselves a disservice.

On the other hand, if we understand and respect learners, we can help them become more effective and better prepare them for a life of learning. When we do so, they are likely to learn more, and to think more highly of their educational program and their instructors. Such learners can offer us more effective criticism of their learning experiences, and help us improve our programs even more. They are also more rewarding to work with, and thereby help us to remain more actively engaged and committed as educators. Finally, some of them will be better prepared to join the ranks of academic medicine, and help to meet the need for first-rate medical educators in the future. One of the best preparations for teaching is to learn with good teachers. By reorienting our focus on the learners, we enhance the overall quality of medical education and practice.

Levels of Understanding

Learners in medicine may grasp knowledge at multiple levels, from the more superficial to the deeper. For example, a term such as "heart failure" might merely indicate that the heart is no longer able to meet the circulatory demands of the body, a definition that is true as far as it goes, or it might imply something much deeper. For example, it might involve an understanding of the etiologies of heart failure, such as chronic hypertension and myocardial ischemia, and it might involve a detailed grasp of the underlying physiology of muscular contraction, including proteins such as myosin and actin. A really sophisticated clinician might add to this an understanding of the common presenting symptoms and signs of heart failure, the various diagnostic tests that might need to be ordered, and the options for therapy. If tomorrow's physicians are to operate with a deep understanding of medicine, we need to cultivate a multidimensional understanding of medicine's most fundamental ideas.

Any time we seek to understand an important medical idea, we can conceive of it in at least four different ways. The modes of understanding might be called the operational, the ostensive, the familial, and the essential. Operational conceptions are perhaps the most straightforward, because they rely on clearly specified criteria. For example, we might say that a patient with a heart rate that exceeds 100 beats/min is tachycardiac, or that a patient whose height is more than two standard deviations below the mean for age suffers from short stature. The emphasis with operational conceptions is on relatively easily observed features that can be compared to normal standards.

Ostensive conceptions, by contrast, also focus on observable features, but attempt to explain an idea by pointing out examples. An ostensive understanding of heart failure would involve recollection of a number of patients who suffered from the disorder. With enough experience, even neophytes can learn to recognize characteristic features of heart failure on history, physical examination, and chest radiography. On a chest radiograph, for example, the heart tends to look enlarged and the lungs appear edematous. Why they appear so is a separate issue.

A third way of understanding is the familial conception, which tries to identify underlying common features that characterize each member of a set of examples to which a particular rubric is applied. For example, there are different types of cardiomyopathy, including dilative, restrictive, and valvular types. Cardiomyopathy is not one thing but many things, and deciding into which group a particular patient's condition falls can be a crucial step in developing an effective therapeutic response. Misunderstanding the category to which a particular case belongs can result in dangerously misdirected therapies, such as treating a patient with a critical valvular stenosis as a case of ischemia, or vice versa.

The deepest level of understanding essential conceptions seeks to integrate surface features with underlying pathophysiological processes. To understand a disease process in essential terms, we must see it not only as a collection of externally observable features, but in terms of deeper concepts. When we understand something in its essence, we can not only identify it, but also understand where it came from and what can be done about it. In this sense, we seek to understand the visible in terms of the invisible, because such pathophysiologic concepts are not— or at least usually not—directly visible. Let us consider each of these levels of understanding in turn.

Operational understanding is probably a reasonable level for novices to aim at, and remains useful even to experts in select situations. For example, if we must merely determine whether a patient's heart rate is above 100 beats/min, the diagnosis of tachycardia becomes relatively apparent and reliable. This gives novices something on which they can immediately hang their hats. This is not to say, however, that experts frequently repair to such conceptions, because they shed relatively little light on what is going on.

Because operational conceptions provide only relatively superficial understanding, they can easily lead us astray. For example, a patient whose heart rate is below 100 beats/min may be very tachycardiac, if the patient has sinus bradycardia and a normal heart rate of only 40 beats/min. Similarly, a heart rate over 100 beats/min may be entirely normal, if the patient is a newborn infant.

All such simple rules have important exceptions that the more seasoned physician must recognize. For example, the chest radiograph can be very deceiving as regards the presence or absence of heart disease. A patient with critical aortic valvular stenosis may have a completely normal chest radiograph. By contrast, a patient whose cardiac silhouette is clearly enlarged may nevertheless have a normal-size heart. Among the mimics of cardiomegaly is underinflation of the lungs, which tends to make the heart appear more short and squat, and pericardial effusion, in which much of the apparent widening of the heart actually represents excess fluid around the heart in the pericardial sac. If we are to make appropriate use of operational approaches to understanding, we need to make sure that learners develop a keen sense of their limitations, and recognize when those limits are reached. For example, we might say that a heart rate of over 100 beats/min is abnormally rapid in adult patients, or that a substantial elevation in heart rate above normal levels can indicate pathologic tachycardia even if it does not reach the 100 beats/min threshold. Likewise, in the case of cardiomegaly on chest radiographs, we need to bear in mind that the chest must be adequately inflated, and that no other factors such as pericardial effusion should be contributing to the apparent width of the heart.

Ostensive conceptions in medicine rely on pattern recognition. To help learners develop stronger ostensive understanding, we might present them with discrimination tasks that ask them to categorize findings as within normal limits or abnormal. For example, we might first show learners photographs of patients with and without exophthalmos, and tell them which patients have the condition and which do not. To help them assess their level of understanding, we might then show them 50 photographs of patients with and without the condition, and ask them to identify which patients appear to have the condition. Over time, learners would tend to become increasingly reliable distinguishers between normal and abnormal findings.

Of course, sole reliance on visual distinguishers can quickly lead learners, as well as practitioners, astray. For example, if medical students are seeking to determine which patients might have hyperthyroidism, they need to look beyond the presence or absence of exophthalmos to other signs of the disorder, such as tachycardia, weight loss, and heat intolerance. Mere pattern recognition is not enough when it comes to categorizing findings and formulating differential diagnoses. To merely recite the same differential diagnosis every time we encounter a particular finding is not enough. We need to learn to seek out other discriminators, such as patient age, the location and duration of the finding, preexisting medical conditions, and aggravating and alleviating factors. We need to use recognizable patterns as a tool, but to supplement them with deeper understanding.

Familial conceptualizations help us to better characterize findings by categorizing them appropriately. Many lesions can lead to enlargement of the heart, and fortunately not all of them enlarge the heart in the same way. On chest radiography, for example, enlargement of the left atrium may cause posterior deviation of the esophagus and a widening of the angle at which the mainstem bronchi branch off from the trachea, whereas a right-sided lesion, such as right atriomegaly, will cause a bulge along the right border of the heart without these other findings.

Exophthalmos from hyperthyroidism is likely to differ quite substantially from that caused by a rhabdomyosarcoma, not least because the former tends to be bilateral and the latter is usually unilateral. Bilateral exophthalmos in patients with pseudotumor will be painful and not associated with tachycardia, whereas bilateral exophthalmos due to hyperthyroidism will tend to be painless and associated with an elevated heart rate.

Essential ways of understanding are both the most illuminating and most difficult of all. Essential understanding moves beyond simple rules of thumb and pattern recognition, and even beyond different schemes for classifying and discriminating findings, to reveal the underlying pathophysiological principles that are at work in them. A relative novice might know that cardiomegaly and pulmonary edema on chest radiography are associated with congestive heart failure. A more experienced observer might look at the same radiograph and eliminate the diagnosis of congestive heart failure, supplanting it with a far more accurate one. For example, suppose the apparent cardiomegaly turns out to be due to a combination of anteroposterior technique and underinflation, whereas the pulmonary edema is nongravity dependent and not associated with pleural effusions. In this situation, acute respiratory distress syndrome might be a far more reasonable diagnosis than congestive heart failure.

By linking findings to underlying pathophysiology, experts are able to enhance their accuracy, precision, and clinical utility. This is because they link the superficial appearance to a deeper understanding of anatomy, physiology, and pathology. The pattern is not the diagnosis in itself. Instead, it is a sign, and one that requires interpretation in the light of more fundamental medical concepts. Mnemonic devices simply will not cut it. To place findings in such a deeper context, it is first necessary to understand pathophysiology. Next the physician needs additional information. In the case of interpreting a chest radiograph, it may be important to know how long the patient has been sick, whether the patient is febrile, whether the patient is in respiratory distress, and the patient's underlying immune status. It is important to make such information available to learners, so that they are not simply making diagnoses from pictures, but taking into account the larger clinical situation. For example, knowing that a patient is immunocompromised may completely change the differential diagnosis in extremely helpful ways.

The goal of distinguishing between these different levels of medical understanding is not to suggest that learners must choose between them, tying their fortunes to one and abandoning the other three. Instead, all four forms have a useful role to play in the practice of medicine. However, the deeper levels of understanding are generally the more powerful, because they provide greater accuracy and reliability, and also do a better job of suggesting additional avenues for further investigation. We need to prepare learners to look beyond what meets the eye to deeper and ultimately invisible levels of knowledge. No one can see congestive heart failure or hyperthyroidism, although the very terms call to mind constellations of physical exam findings and diagnostic test results.

One way to assess the depth of learners' understanding is to question them about what they see. Are they thinking about it in simple rules of thumb, or are they repairing to deeper essential concepts that underlie what is before them? What questions do they pose? Are they making creative inferences based on analysis at the essential level of conceptualization, or are they merely determining whether A looks like B or C? Ultimately, we want learners to construct narratives of what they encounter, attempting to put together all four levels of understanding, and especially the deepest ones, in a single integrated story.

Testing, Testing

Today's premedical and medical students are brought up on a steady diet of tests, an observation that applies to a lesser degree to residents, as well. Because tests play such a large role in defining the intellectual agendas of these learners, it is vital that we examine the tests we administer to ensure that they promote the professional health of those they are evaluating. Premedical students, medical students, and residents spend hundreds, even thousands of hours preparing for these tests, and it is vital that we look carefully at the examinations themselves to determine their professional impact. No test is perfect, and opportunities may exist to engineer the tests to better foster the development of the sorts of physician we hope to be educating.

Tests can play two fundamentally different roles. The first is an evaluative role. We give learners tests to determine whether they are learning what they are supposed to be learning, to determine how well they are learning it, and to determine who is learning it well and who not so well. In other words, testing functions in part to sort and select students. For example, we use standardized tests to evaluate medical school applicants, and we also assess residency candidates based in part on their examination scores. The other function of testing is a formative one, a function too often neglected in medical education. This use of testing capitalizes on the fact that learners will try hardest to learn the things on which they expect to be tested. If we take this function seriously, we can not only determine who is learning the most and who is not learning enough, we can also shape the learning objectives of all learners. Of course, testing is not the only form of evaluation, and there may be some educational objectives, such as those pertaining to professionalism, that do not lend themselves well to testing but some other form of assessment.

We must guard against the temptation to regard the examinations themselves as the learning objective. The test is just a tool, a means of determining what learning has taken place. The goal is knowledge and skill, to which the test is a means. We cannot make students more knowledgeable merely by testing them, any more than we can fatten cattle by weighing them. On the other hand, there is no question that most of us probably studied longer and harder in our collegiate and medical school courses in part because the prospect of a test loomed before us. We need to ask, then, how do our examinations do a good job of evaluating, and where do opportunities for improvement exist? Do our examinations foster an appropriate vision of professional excellence?

In beginning to critically examine our examinations, we need to consider the many roles they play beyond selecting and sorting learners and motivating study. For one thing, every test we administer to medical students and residents represents a form of fiduciary professional self-regulation. We are in effect certifying that medical students and residents have demonstrated a sufficient level of proficiency in basic areas to move on to the next stage of their training, and ultimately, to practice independently. If the profession does not regulate its own ranks and attempt to identify, remediate, and perhaps ultimately discharge prospective physicians who are not performing at an adequate level, communities will have no choice but to do so themselves. Medicine and its educators must live up to the responsibility to ensure a minimal level of competence in those we advance.

Our examinations also have the potential to elevate the general level of practice. As new developments come to light that can benefit patients, we can ensure that they are incorporated into training programs, including their evaluative activities. By changing the content of examinations, in other words, we can change what medical students and residents are attempting to learn, and thereby enhance the general level of knowledge and skill in the medical community. This is not to suggest that examination writers bear primary responsibility for keeping the profession moving forward. It is inevitable that the content of examinations will lag behind the latest scientific and clinical developments. However, the content of our examinations need not and should not remain the same year after year, decade after decade, or we will exert a retarding influence on medicine that redounds to no one's benefit.

Another opportunity for sparking improvement through examinations is to encourage learners to pursue innovative alternative professional pathways. There is a tendency for medical education to be a process of homogenization, turning out graduates who are similar to one another than they were when they began. Certainly this is desirable with respect to basic knowledge and skills, but we also need to encourage diversity in the profession and enable learners to develop their distinctive interests and abilities. For example, some learners might choose to explore an interest in research, and we might allow them to take examinations that are more research focused. Others might choose pathways in education, leadership, or service. We need to develop the next generation of researchers, educators, leaders, and professional servants, but if learners who would otherwise develop such interests are inhibited from doing so merely because they believe they must perform well on the same clinical examinations as everyone else, we may stunt their development, to the detriment of the profession and the patients it serves.

Another use of examinations is to foster the development of professional competencies beyond those usually tested in courses and board examinations. For example, merely knowing a lot is not enough. To function effectively as a physician, we need to communicate what we know to other physicians, health professionals, and above all, patients and families. How effectively do learners convey the urgency of findings, and what systems would they put in place to ensure that urgent or unexpected findings do not "slip through the cracks?" How well are we preparing our learners for a lifetime of self-directed study? How well are they able to critically evaluate the professional literature, determining where conclusions are scientifically justified or not? And how well are they prepared to critically evaluate their own practices, to treat the everyday practice of medicine as a learning opportunity for themselves and their patients? These are competencies that creative examinations can help foster.

We also need to critically examine our tests to determine whether they are focusing learners' attention on the most fundamental and practically relevant material before them. Poor examinations can lead learners to expend great effort committing to memory minutiae and esoterica that bear little relevance to the opportunities they will face as clinicians, researchers, educators, and leaders. The net that our examinations cast need not be so wide that it leaves learners feeling that they are responsible for knowing everything. What do they really need to know, and what do they merely need to know how to find out? We need to conceptualize learners less as repositories of information and more as knowledge seekers, who will use the core of knowledge they acquire during their training to guide both their practice and their further learning. What really needs to be in that core?

We need to point out explicitly to learners that preparing for examinations is not their only responsibility, and that some of the most important lessons they will learn will never be tested in a formal sense. How, for example, do we learn how to talk with patients, or how to handle disappointment? We need to keep the examinations in perspective, so that these other lessons are not drowned in a sea of test-fever. Other systems of evaluation need to be in place, and learners need to be aware of them. The goal of medical education is not to prepare for and pass all the tests, but to prepare to be a good physician. A medical student who shuns as much patient interaction as possible so as to have more time to study for the final examination is making a mistake, and we need systems of evaluation robust enough to detect and remediate such misplaced priorities.

A major function of our examinations that we rarely think about is their role as a rite of passage. Anthropologists have shed considerable light on such rituals, which include a rigorous course of preparation, acquisition of complex knowledge and skills, a risk-laden trial or performance, and unreserved acceptance of individuals who have successfully negotiated the course. The high-stakes tests that divide up medical education serve these same functions, and play an important role in the psychological and social lives of our learners. When can they say, "Enough!" and know that they have made it? Passing such examinations makes them feel that they have proved themselves, and that they are becoming full-fledged members of the profession.

We should not pretend that learner performance on examinations provides an accurate prediction of their eventual level of excellence as physicians. The capacity of standardized tests to make such predictions is the subject of intense skepticism on the part of many professional educators. Perhaps the most famous test of all, the SAT, once known as the Scholastic Aptitude Test, is now known simply as the SAT, because the Educational Testing Service in Princeton, New Jersey recognized that it is not really a measure of scholastic aptitude. To be sure, learners who fail examinations may be telling us something important: that they are not making enough of an effort, that they do not know how to study effectively, that something else is happening in their lives, and so on. Yet practicing medicine is much more than taking tests, and we need to bear that limitation in mind in assessing the performance of our learners on standardized tests. Darwin and Einstein, for example, were notoriously mediocre students.

We should remind learners that in a few years, no one will either care or even know how well they scored on most of the tests they take. Patients and colleagues do not check up on physicians' examination scores, and everyone who wears a white coat is known as "doctor," regardless of where they graduated in their medical school class. Nor do we allocate research funds, choose the best educators, or assign positions of leadership on the basis of test scores. We recognize that other traits and spheres of performance are more germane to such choices. Passing an examination is not, and should never be, mistaken for the crowning achievement of a physician's life.

In conclusion, several steps are in order. First, we should encourage all learners to spend less time worrying about their examinations and more time becoming the best physicians they can be. The two are not always coextensive. Second, we should try to bring our examinations more in line with what we think makes a good physician, so that time and energy spent on examination preparation redound to the greatest possible benefit to the profession. Third, we should ensure that our examinations are not dominated by the arcane and abstruse, and focus instead on what learners most need to know. Fourth, we should ensure that learners receive comprehensive and formative evaluations that address those crucial aspects of development that are not easily tested. The next generation of physicians deserves an even more appealing and nutritional educational diet.

Teaching Medical Students

If we are to provide medical students with the best possible education, we need to study the features of educational success. These features include providing students with clear objectives, enabling them to function as members of a team, granting them substantial control over their success or failure, offering them constructive feedback, providing them challenging learning tasks, and allowing them to contribute meaningfully to patient care.

Learning objectives are a powerful tool for enhancing educational outcomes. If students have no targets in view, their learning will be compromised. Some medical students may find it difficult to formulate well-informed learning objectives for themselves. In some cases, the only explicit learning objectives students receive are reading assignments. Although better than no objectives, reading assignments merely tell students where they are expected to learn, and provide no idea what they should be able to do as a result. Moreover, mere reading assignments often leave students wondering if readings comprise the only source from which they are expected to learn. Does this imply that clinical time with practicing physicians is unlikely to provide any worthwhile learning opportunities? Many students organize their learning around what they expect to be tested on, and it is important to ensure that the full range of learning experiences is represented in learning objectives and evaluation techniques. A common requirement is attendance. Students are expected to attend lectures, and to be present on the clinical service to which they are assigned.

However, merely showing up is a rather low-level goal. Medical educators should make sure that the time students spend in clinical departments is put to good use. To help students come away from clinical experiences with more than merely a perfect attendance record, it is important to help them understand what they are expected to learn when they are there. A simple list of learning objectives would often suffice. Despite Woody Allen's adage that 90% of life is simply showing up, we sell students short if we fail to help them define clearly what they should be doing while they are with us.

We could ask students to carry out independent learning tasks as individuals or members of groups. For example, students might develop case write-ups to be used in educating other students. They could be challenged to make meaningful contributions to the clinical work of a department, by assuming responsibility for helping to work up particular cases. Ideally, the learning associated with such projects would be especially useful in the medical specialty they plan to enter. Such projects would enable them to avoid the kind of superficial learning that is a mile wide and only an inch deep, by spending part of their time delving more deeply into topics of particular interest to them.

Perhaps one of the greatest opportunities before medical educators is to define teams to which students belong. When third- and fourth-year medical students are on rotations such as internal medicine or surgery, they function as team players with defined roles. The team consists of an attending physician, a senior resident, a junior resident, and one or more medical students. In many cases, this team remains together throughout the course of a month-long experience, allowing members to get to know one another and work together to accomplish a shared mission.

More of medical education could emulate this model. When students are asked during their surgery rotation whose team they are on, they provide an immediate response. Asked the same question during some other phases of their medical school career, they may respond, "What team?" Instead of contributing, they may feel that they are merely imposing on the faculty members and residents to whom they are assigned.

Medical education is not only a cognitive process, it is also a social process. Students' appraisals of their educational experiences take into account more than simply how much they learned from books and lectures. To address this problem, educators should look for opportunities to enable medical students to function as team members. For example, students might be placed in small groups with defined educational goals, such as developing 15 min group presentations for their fellow medical students. Each student might be assigned not to a particular clinical service, but to a particular resident, with whom they would be expected to work throughout their time in a course. They might contribute by helping to work up cases where additional clinical information is needed. Such an experience would provide students with more of a sense of camaraderie, and residents with a more clearly defined role as educators.

As performance-oriented people with high expectations for their own achievement, medical students need to feel that they exercise control over how they perform. If the whole evaluation process is a mystery to them, their motivation will be undermined, and they are more likely to find their educational experience unsatisfactory. This can compromise student evaluations of teaching faculty, reduce student interest in courses, and discourage students from pursuing particular specialties as careers. In cases where students are interacting with a shifting cast of residents and staff, they may wonder whether meaningful evaluation is even possible, particularly if most of the people they work with do not know their name. Students may question what they can do to enhance their performance, other than simply show up every day and project a positive mental attitude.

Most courses could evaluate students in multiple dimensions, which should be clearly mapped out. A potentially valuable educational strategy would be to invite students to participate in determining their grade. For example, students might have the option of completing a project as part of their grade. In schools with competency-based curricula, each specialty might provide students an opportunity to demonstrate one or more competencies. Where possible, students should be furnished with examples of excellent, good, and poor performances, including samples of past students' work.

For some students, a course in a discipline serves as an important opportunity to explore a career option. Special opportunities might be made available to such students, including the opportunity to meet with a faculty advisor to learn more about the field. Highly motivated students, especially those aspiring to a particular specialty, may welcome the opportunity to do a special project as a means of distinguishing themselves as residency candidates.

Failure to receive feedback is one of the most de-motivating experiences to which highly achievement-oriented people can be subjected. Conversely, providing more frequent and higher-quality feedback is an excellent way of improving students' overall impression of a course and the people who teach it. Timing is an important aspect of good feedback. There is a tendency for medical school courses to base students' grades on a single written exam scheduled at the end of the course. Likewise, written feedback from faculty members typically becomes available only after a course has concluded. These practices make it very difficult for students to use feedback constructively. It is as though basketball players learned only at the end of the game whether any of their shots had gone through the hoop.

An ideal system of feedback would provide learners with actionable suggestions on a weekly or even daily basis. To achieve such an objective may require the introduction of computer-based instruction to avoid overburdening faculty. Perhaps even more important, faculty members should get into the habit of incorporating constructive feedback into their daily routines. One means of doing so would be to make a point of asking frequent questions to the students on clinical services, to determine if they are truly learning the principles discussed in readings and lectures. Some questions might even be repeated from day to day, to ensure that they are retaining what they have learned. Even more important is to give students a chance to apply what they are learning to clinical care.

All courses need to present students with meaningful challenges. Assigning learning tasks to fourth-year students that one would normally provide to first year students is a mistake, because the more experienced students find such tasks insufficiently challenging and lose interest. Likewise, assigning fourth-year students learning tasks that one would normally provide fourth-year residents can prove equally de-motivating, because the less experienced learners do not know where to start, find the task overwhelming, and give up.

The appropriate level of challenge is not an absolute quantity but a relative one, which needs to be tailored to the learner. On the other hand, there are absolute principles. For example, no learner at any level will find it challenging to sit quietly, merely struggling to feign interest and remain awake throughout a long monologue. Likewise, simply seeing how many facts students can recall from assigned readings provides a relatively low-level challenge. Better challenges require students not merely to recall information but to synthesize what they know, draw distinctions, and solve problems.

A top-notch course will invite medical students to test themselves as physicians. For example, they might be asked to look up the results of laboratory studies, to review medical records, and to speak with other physicians involved in the care of particular patients, in an effort to help determine what test to perform, what differential diagnosis to offer, and what further evaluation to recommend. Top-notch students can perform an important educational function in a department, by reminding faculty members and residents of information they have forgotten, and helping them remain abreast of new developments in medicine. There is no reason that students should not be invited to play the role of instructor from time to time, or that faculty members should fail to benefit from what they know.

Perhaps the single greatest opportunity in the curricula of many departments, particularly in courses for advanced medical students, is to get students involved in helping to care for patients. As soon as possible, in medical training, students should take histories and perform physical examinations. They should track down the results of diagnostic testing and request consultations from other clinical services. They should learn to perform procedures, such as phlebotomy and lumbar punctures, and their contributions should form a part of the patient's permanent medical record, helping to spare the time and energy of other members on the team. They should also make presentations to their teams and help to educate patients.

To a medical student, few experiences are more invigorating than acting as a doctor, and that means actually getting to do some of the things that doctors do. They can help to educate patients about diagnostic tests and therapeutic procedures and assist in their performance. In every course, we should strive to enable students to learn things that they regard as directly relevant to patient care. What skills will students need every day during their internships, and how can we incorporate them into the curriculum from the outset? Through the judicious use of new educational technology and careful planning of the curriculum, the evaluation process, and teacher scheduling, the costs of improving medical student education can be minimized. The overarching goal of educational reform should be to transform medical students from passive observers to active participants, whose contributions are both welcomed and appreciated.

5

Educational Excellence

You can tell whether a man is clever by his answers. You can tell whether he is wise by his questions.

Naguib Mahfouz, *Khufu's Wisdom*

Worthy of Emulation

Many of the most important lessons in the education of physicians are not well conveyed by lectures, books, and electronic media. These lessons touch on such topics as work ethic, goal setting, patient interaction, consultation, and coping with uncertainty and failure. Whether we are aware of it or not, each medical educator manifests characteristic patterns of conduct in these areas, and these habits exert a formative influence on medical students, residents, and other learners. It is a mistake to conceptualize learning as the mere memorization of facts. It also involves the adoption of attitudes and patterned approaches to daily work, and this adoption often takes place at a subconscious level.

In reflecting back over our careers, many of us can easily call to mind a few individuals whose habits of practice exerted a particularly formative influence on our own development, people who stand out as role models. One of the most rewarding experiences for any medical educator is to see learners incorporate elements of our style into their own approach to practice. Needless to say, if the attitude or conduct is a poor one, this can also prove one of the most mortifying of experiences. In either case, however, medical educators need to pay more attention to emulation.

As we have seen, emulation can take one of two fundamentally different forms: constructive or destructive. Constructive emulation occurs when learners adopt attitudes and patterns of conduct that enable them to perform better as physicians. For example, a resident may, as a result of working with a particularly well-organized faculty physician, develop the habit of taking a few minutes each morning to outline key objectives for the workday. A resident who does so is more likely to be productive than one who does not, and this could be one of the most important lessons the resident learns over many years of training.

By contrast, destructive emulation occurs when learners adopt habits that undermine their excellence. Consider a disgruntled and frankly cynical faculty

R.B. Gunderman, *Achieving Excellence in Medical Education,* DOI: 10.1007/978-0-85729-307-7_5, © Springer-Verlag London Limited 2011 member, whose residents tend to develop such habits as criticizing colleagues behind their backs, thereby corroding collegiality and mutual respect within the department. One goal of all medical educators should be to cultivate opportunities for constructive emulation and reduce opportunities for destructive emulation. We need to consider not only the content of the formal curriculum, but that of the informal and even hidden curriculum, as well. With whom are learners working, and to what effect? One way of enhancing our educational effectiveness as role models is to strengthen our understanding of this vital but often overlooked aspect of education.

First, we must recognize that each one of us, whether we are on the faculty or not, is a role model. Peers and even subordinates influence how learners develop. For example, residents learn many of their most important lessons from other residents, and medical students learn many of their most important lessons from other medical students. I have certainly learned a great deal from residents and medical students I worked with as a faculty member. Once we become aware that our conduct exerts a wider influence than our formal authority might suggest, we can take better care to ensure that we are projecting a worthy image. We do not cease being educators the second we walk out the classroom door, and some non-faculty colleagues exert even greater formative influence than some members of the faculty. For example, medical students frequently learn more about how to be a physician from the house staff than from the faculty.

What are the functions of people whose attitudes and conduct constitute a worthy example for others? First, they reinforce and augment constructive behavior in others. A medical student's commitment to communicating well with patients is strengthened by working with a physician who places a high priority on effective communication. Second, the conduct of good role models tends to inhibit the development of destructive patterns of conduct. A medical student who witnesses a resident remain calm in circumstances where many others would have lost their cool glimpses firsthand the benefits of keeping one's temper in check. Such experiences send the subtle but important message that abusive behavior is simply not okay. Third, learners emulate new habits that make them better physicians. When we offer a good example of how to obtain informed consent for medical procedures, learners are more likely to do it well themselves.

For learners to grow and develop as excellent physicians as least three conditions must be met. First, learners need to be paying attention to their role models. Potential role models who are not even noticed are unlikely to exert much influence. Similarly, role models who are regarded as irrelevant because they are viewed as insufficiently engaged are unlikely to offer much. To be an effective role model, we need to be close to learners and actively exhibiting attitudes and patterns of conduct to which learners need to attend. We also need to be credible and worthy of emulation. If our clinical skills are perceived as inadequate, learners will not look up to us. Finally, learners must not have definite and inflexible attitudes toward what we do. If they think they already know everything, they are unlikely to benefit from working side by side with us. We need to afford learners an opportunity to recognize what they do not know, to appreciate its importance, and to interact with individuals who exhibit the appropriate attitudes and patterns of conduct.

One area in which we can provide an important example to learners is clarity about goals. If medical students, residents, and even colleagues do not see clearly what they are trying to learn, they are unlikely to seize important learning opportunities. The problem is not that these learners are unmotivated or unintelligent. They simply do not know what they are trying to learn, and as a result, learn less than they could. By helping learners develop a clearer sense of purpose, we can help them learn more. We can help them by modeling how we form our own learning objectives and structuring our own workday so that we are always trying to learn.

Two types of consequences affect learner performance. One type of consequence is vicarious, and the other self-generated. We learn vicariously when we see the consequences that accrue to other learners. For example, if we see a colleague publicly humiliated because of an incorrect response, we may become less inclined to volunteer to answer questions ourselves. This is not to say that all criticism is bad. Failure to point out mistakes can be even worse, and criticism can definitely exert a salutary effect, as long as it encourages learners to improve their performance and provides guidance on how to do so. We need to bear in mind that the way we treat a learner affects not only that individual, but others as well. Even interactions that are not directly witnessed by others are often rapidly spread through informal channels of communication. In some cases, particularly memorable accounts may be passed down from year to year and even generation to generation, becoming part of the folklore of our educational programs.

Self-generated consequences are equally important. These arise independent of the social environment. In some cases, we may modify our attitude and conduct based on our own self-reflection, independent of criticism or praise from others. If we are to become excellent physicians, we need to develop this talent for self-examination, so that we can regulate our own professional trajectory based on our internal moral compass. This provides a more powerful and enduring bulwark against destructive conduct than fear of detection, humiliation, or punishment. By sharing our self-examination with learners and encouraging them to pay attention to their own internal compasses, we can help them to develop fully as excellent physicians.

To highlight the best habits of physicians, we should seek out opportunities to incorporate them into the formal curriculum. We need to make clear to learners that their ethics is no less important than their fund of knowledge and clinical skills. One way to implement this is to ensure that we take character into account in our selection and evaluation processes for medical students and residents. When done well, such programs highlight the importance of character in medicine, provide some encouragement for exemplary conduct, and help to foster the development of constructive internal goals and standards.

One way to foster the quality of emulation in our educational programs is to develop formal mentorship responsibilities. The term mentor is derived from an elderly character in Homer's *Odyssey*, who serves as a friend and advisor to Odysseus (Fig. 5.1). A mentor is less a teacher than a confidante, role model, and coach. A mentor can serve as a quasi-official representative of the informal curriculum, giving learners someone to call on when they need counsel in the face of uncertainty. Mentorship often works best in an informal environment, such as a

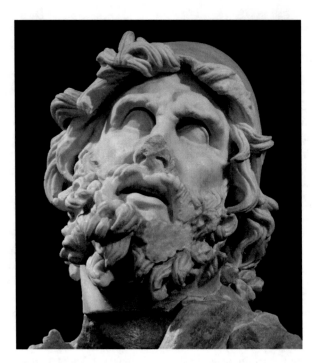

Fig. 5.1 Head of Odysseus from a second century marble statue. As the background to Homer's epics the *Iliad* and the *Odyssey*, Odysseus reluctantly leaves to fight alongside the Greeks in the Trojan war, a venture from which he will not return for 20 years. Before he leaves, he asks his friend Mentor to watch over his son and his household. Later the goddess Athena appears to both Odysseus and his son in the guise of Mentor, encouraging the latter to stand up for what is right and go out in search of his father. The term mentor has come to mean a trusted teacher and advisor (Courtesy of Wikimedia Commons)

meal, where learners may feel more comfortable about raising such issues as interpersonal conflict, balancing personal and professional life, and choosing between different career paths. What difficult decisions have we faced, how did we cope with them, and what did we learn as a result? It is probably wise for learners to have at least two mentors, one on the faculty and one from a slightly more advanced peer group.

We must guard against implicitly encouraging learners to develop an aversion to challenge. It is all too easy for many learners to develop such a fear of failure that they begin to avoid new things. If learners never see us try something new, and never get to see how we handle disappointment, they may develop the disabling view that they, too, should never take risks. If they see us always avoiding failure and covering it up whenever it occurs, they may fail to develop their own ways of coping with and learning from disappointments. Overconfidence is certainly problematic, and we want learners to develop a healthy respect for their own limitations. To foster a willingness to venture into uncharted territory, we need to challenge learners in ways that stretch them beyond their comfort zone yet hold out a reasonable probability of success, so that they develop their sense of personal efficacy. We want learners to regard heightened tension as an opportunity to excel, not a signal to give up.

We need to exemplify how we construct our own scenarios of success. We need to share with learners how we use our time to imagine our goals and visualize ourselves achieving them. Less successful people tend not to have a clear vision of their own goals, and even if they do, they cannot foresee a path by which to reach them. They tend to set lower goals for themselves, expend less effort in their pursuit, and give up more easily when they encounter obstacles. People with a higher sense of personal efficacy tend to analyze new situations in light of their goals and devote considerable energy to developing strategies by which to excel. They aim higher, work harder, and persist longer when faced with obstacles. By encouraging learners to discuss and reflect on their own visions of success and the routes by which they might pursue them, we can increase their ability to fashion rewarding careers for themselves.

Throughout most of medical education, the evaluation of learners is heavily biased in favor of information recall. We tend to evaluate medical students and residents by what they can remember. This bias reflects the fact that it is relatively easy to determine whether learners can recall a particular fact. By contrast, a learner's approach to unfamiliar situations is much more difficult to detect, describe, and measure. Despite this challenge, we need to develop evaluation systems that extend beyond what is easiest to measure, and encompass what is most important to learn as well. We need to pay attention to motivation, confidence, self-reflection, and self-regulation of learning. If we do not, learners are likely to achieve less than their potential. To what degree are we assessing our own performance on parameters other than fund of knowledge, and how well are we sharing this perspective with learners?

Above all, it is vital that we bring to the arena of medical education sound characters, high standards of professional conduct, and a deep commitment to the welfare of our patients, our colleagues, and our institutions. Learners need to see that we care about these matters, because they are not only developing their diagnostic and therapeutic acumen, they are also developing their professional character. It is equally important that we guard against hypocrisy. If we constantly chafe about the need to give lectures or publish papers, how seriously will our trainees contemplate academic careers, no matter how much lip service we pay to their importance? Our profession cannot afford to juxtapose heavenly words and subterranean conduct.

Performance Appraisal

Each of us is influenced, at times powerfully influenced, by the performance appraisals we receive. Learners rely to a great extent on the appraisals of people we respect to determine whether we are performing at a satisfactory level. The absence of a timely, clear, and constructive program of performance appraisal is a black mark against any educational program. Conversely, a good performance appraisal system represents an important teaching strategy that can offer immense benefit to both learners and educators. Despite these advantages, however, many of us do not employ performance appraisal as effectively as we might. If we can improve our performance in this area, we can achieve important improvements in the overall quality of our educational program.

Every medical student and resident education program is required to provide performance appraisals of learners in order to retain its accreditation. Yet many learners lament that the appraisals they receive are too infrequent, too unclear, or too unhelpful. This probably stems, in part, from the fact that most medical educators have received little training in the evaluative component of education. Another difficulty with evaluation in the current medical education environment is that faculty members are under increasing pressure to enhance their clinical productivity, which can make performance appraisal both more difficult and more expensive. We feel that we are simply too busy to devote much time and energy to this aspect of medical education. In some cases, we regard evaluation as a burden we would rather not shoulder, and shirk it when we can.

Performance appraisal is not merely a means of culling out unsatisfactory learners or giving learners a pat on the back. Properly understood, it is one of the most important opportunities we enjoy to enhance learning. It can help both learners and educators perform at a higher level, and thereby enhance the educational rewards of both. On the other hand, if we do not do it well, both learners and educators learn to dread it. We need to review some of the key principles of effective performance appraisal, and thereby enhance our performance in this important area.

One weakness of many educational programs is the dearth of serious performance appraisal, particularly in the residency and fellowship phases of medical education. It may lead learners to the false conclusion that "no news is good news," or it may create the even more serious misimpression that no one really cares how learners perform. I have heard many learners express the view that they are operating in a near vacuum, where they function for weeks or even months without any meaningful appraisal of the work they are doing. It is reasonable for every learner to expect to receive formal and informal evaluations on a frequent basis. It is also entirely reasonable for learners to request an appraisal of their performance. Good learners want to know what educators regard as their strengths and weaknesses, and what they could do to augment the former and redress the latter.

One obstacle to performance appraisal may be educators' aversion to criticism. Some of us may wish to avoid criticizing or contradicting learners, perhaps because we fear that they will like us less or give us poorer evaluations as educators. Yet failing to correct a misapprehension represents tacit support for correctable misunderstanding, which is antithetical to our educational mission. As educators, we have a moral responsibility to let our learners know when they have gotten something wrong, particularly if it is an error that might someday harm someone. We cannot let our penchant for being regarded as "nice guys" interfere with our duties as educators who are dedicated to the promotion of understanding.

There are more and less effective ways of pointing out mistakes. One ineffective approach is criticism that verges on sadism, where every misstep is seized upon as an opportunity to loose the dogs of humiliation and intimidation. Another more benign type of criticism may be almost equally ineffective because it merely finds fault without providing any constructive guidance for improvement. Effective performance appraisal provides, or perhaps better yet fosters, real insight. It is possible to cushion criticism by also pointing to something the learner has done well. Malicious evaluations only poison the educational environment by creating resentment and even anger, disrupting the development of a respectful and trusting relationship.

We need to be secure enough in our own professional competence that we do not need to bring learners down a peg or two just to feel comfortable with our own performance. Instead of putting learners in their place, we need to form partnerships with learners to help them better define appropriate learning expectations, identify deficiencies or at least opportunities for improvement, and offer appreciation and praise where it is deserved. The fact that we as educators may receive less performance appraisal than we would like is no license to treat learners the same way. We especially need to guard against the tendency to provide only negative evaluations. We should try equally hard to let learners know they have done a good job and thank them for their help.

Although we have a responsibility to let learners know when they have misunderstood something, we have an equally important responsibility to help them become better appraisers of their own performance. They will not be students or trainees forever, and they will not always have faculty members watching over them. We want learners to regard their practice reflectively and even self-critically, so that they are always striving to learn from their experience. If we treat every request for evaluation or clarification as an opportunity to blame learners for failing to know, they may develop a counterproductive fear of recognizing and admitting what they do not know. This is a sure prescription for overlooking opportunities to improve. We never want learners to develop the view that their survival depends on never getting caught not knowing something.

Good questions are ultimately more important to our profession than good answers, because it is our ability to contribute to new discoveries that will shape the future of the field. When we are surrounded by learners who are good at asking questions, our own practice is enriched through more intense self-examination. We often discover that we do not understand matters as well as we suppose. Often the best response to a good question is not the right answer, but another good question, encouraging learners to investigate the matter for themselves. We need to foster learners' inner sense of what it means to understand something well, and to recognize what steps to take to achieve a deeper grasp of the question at hand.

We want learners to pay careful attention to their own learning performance, and to seek out opportunities to improve the quality of their work. The problem may be a simple one, such as the failure to devote enough time to study, or failure to study in an effective way. We want them to benefit from the educator's point of view, but to develop their own point of view as well, which may not always be the same as our own. In the final analysis, the best indicator of learner performance may not be how much we know, but how much we are able to learn, and what we are able to make of that understanding. Both formal and informal evaluations can help promote this objective, and warrant more attention than many of us have been paying to them.

Developing Educators

The ongoing investments of medical schools in their faculty members' capabilities as clinicians and researchers should be accompanied by ongoing investments in their capabilities as teachers. Part of the promise of faculty development stems from the fact that most medical educators have received little or no formal instruction in how to teach. The curricula of our medical schools and residency programs frequently ignore teaching, and we tend to make the unwarranted assumption that anyone who has completed medical school and residency is a qualified educator. In fact, however, educational researchers have shed considerable light on what makes an effective teacher, and departments and schools can capitalize on these discoveries by developing faculty development programs.

The quality of today's healthcare bears the imprint of the medical educators who have taught medicine over the past few decades, and the way medicine is being taught today will influence the quality of healthcare for decades to come. If medicine is poorly taught, the quality of healthcare will suffer. If it is taught well, everyone involved in healthcare stands to benefit, including not only patients and physicians, but families, allied health professionals, employers, and healthcare payers. The same can be said for the quality of biomedical research. Producing top-notch biomedical researchers requires top-notch research training programs, which in turn require top-notch research faculties.

Many crucial educational decisions are powerfully influenced by the medical school faculty, including who is admitted to medical school and residency, what gets taught there, and how learners are evaluated. In public education, teacher quality—as measured by education, experience, and test scores on licensing examinations—has been shown to have a greater impact on student achievement than any other single factor. In short, the quality of medical practice hinges on the quality of the people teaching medicine.

Despite the huge influence of medical education over the future of medicine, education has not fared well over the past decade or two. The rise of managed care has spurred academic health centers to devote more and more attention to the generation of clinical revenue. Faced with declining levels of reimbursement for care provided in academic centers, many department chairs and deans have adopted policies that encourage their faculty to behave more like community physicians. Each hour that a medical school faculty member devotes to teaching represents an hour of lost clinical revenue, which some see as placing the academic health center at a competitive disadvantage. Yet time spent in delivering more clinical care clearly generates more revenue. Research, too, offers opportunities to generate additional income, through extramural funding and partnerships with industry. Devoting more time to education, however, usually generates no additional income.

As a result, education begins to look to a healthcare administrator like a loss leader, a product on which merchants will tolerate a loss in hopes of attracting customers who will more than make up the difference with other purchases. Far from inspiring enthusiasm, medical education has become a business line in which many administrators feel less and less inclined to invest. If we regard the traditional structure of academic medicine as a tripod made up of legs of clinical care, research, and education, then education has become the short leg. If we neglect education too much, the whole enterprise may topple over.

To meet these challenges, it is vital that academic health centers develop creative strategies for maintaining and strengthening their educational missions. Healthcare payers seeking cost reductions are unlikely to take up this fight on their own. Instead, department chairs and faculty members must demonstrate that high-quality medical education represents a good investment, and develop innovative strategies for funding it. Central to any such efforts is a reexamination of the core values of medical education, including those components of the educational enterprise where new investments are most likely to pay off. If we want to raise the bar of medical education to a new level, where can we best invest our time and energies?

As a rule, physicians set high standards for themselves and become frustrated when they are unable to perform at a high level. Some individuals are naturally gifted and would do a good job in almost any situation, but, most of us tend to perform better when we understand what we are doing. By helping faculty members better understand effective teaching, we can improve their teaching performance, and thereby enhance their sense of professional satisfaction. This is especially important at a time when many academic disciplines are having difficulty recruiting and retaining physicians in academic careers.

Another benefit is the positive impact of faculty development efforts on morale. Laboring under ever greater pressure to sustain and augment clinical throughput, many faculty members have become discouraged about their academic missions. Some chose academic careers in part because they liked to teach, and as managed care has eroded institutional enthusiasm for education, more and more of them have left academic medicine entirely. If the tide of disenchantment and demoralization is to be turned, it is important for academic health centers to begin demonstrating a renewed commitment to teaching excellence.

By investing in faculty development programs, academic departments can provide a much needed demonstration of their commitment to education. What topics should be included in a top-notch faculty development program for academic physicians? One crucial topic is curriculum development. At the level of medical student teaching, what do medical students really need to learn about our disciplines? Is residency primarily about transmitting facts, or should a greater role be played by the cultivation of newer capabilities, such as critical thinking, interpersonal communication, and research methodology? One of the greatest benefits of reexamining the curriculum of any educational enterprise is the fact that it gets faculty members talking to one another again about the nature of their educational mission, including their differing conceptions of what makes an excellent physician.

Aside from *what* should be taught, reexamination of the curriculum also spawns discussion of *how* it should be taught. Are didactic lectures the best way to teach? Should residents be expected to learn mostly on their own through independent study? What role should computer-based tutorial learning play? To a large degree, how to teach depends on what we are trying to get across.

If a residency program determines that critical thinking is a skill to which it needs to devote more attention, making use of a pedagogical technique such as problem-based learning might warrant consideration. Problem-based learning has become quite popular in medical school curricula, because it encourages students to learn through actively solving problems, rather than passively receiving information. For example, instead of giving first-year residents a series of lectures on diagnostic imaging, a faculty member might present them with a case of a patient with right upper quadrant pain, and ask them to assess the advantages and disadvantages of various imaging modalities in the workup.

Another important topic for the curriculum of a faculty development course is learning theory. What is known about how young adults learn, and what steps can be taken to create a better fit between instructional approaches and the psychology of learning? Many of us know very little about cognitive psychology, but we each operate from an implicit notion of how learners learn. For example, it makes a huge difference in teaching whether we regard residents as empty vessels to be filled up with facts or as active inquirers who need to be given chances to investigate. By examining some of the most prominent learning theories, medical educators can develop a better understanding of learning, both our students' and their own.

Another important lesson of learning theory is the fact that not all learners are created equal. For example, different people tend to learn better in different formats. Some learn best in the context of group interaction and others in independent study. Some learn best when they read information and others when they hear it. In recognizing that such differences exist, educators can take care to employ multiple instructional strategies, thereby giving every learner a chance to do his or her best.

Another key topic in a curriculum of faculty development is educational assessment. Students tend to learn what they expect to be evaluated on, which means that the choice of educational assessment strategies powerfully affects where their focus lies. For example, if residents believe that they will be evaluated primarily on the basis of their fund of knowledge, they will spend much of their time studying textbooks and review manuals. If they believe that clinical skills are paramount, they will focus on those. On the other hand, if they believe that critical thinking, communication, and research skills will not show up on any tests or evaluation forms, they will tend to neglect them.

There are major questions in educational assessment. For example, which is more important for assessment to focus on, teacher effectiveness or learner outcomes? Teacher effectiveness focuses on what the teacher is doing. An example of a teacher effectiveness measure would be peer review of teaching. Another would be teacher evaluation forms filled out by students or residents. Because there is so little peer review of teaching, most teacher evaluation has come to be heavily learner driven, meaning that the only formal evaluations and rewards for teaching are based on learner assessments. Whether peer assessment of teaching would produce the same assessments is unknown, but there is a danger that educators may begin to behave as though we were trying to win a popularity contest. If the only evaluation of my teaching is based on what students have to say, over time I may feel subtle pressure to give students better evaluations, in hopes of getting better evaluations myself.

By contrast, learner outcome-based assessment means that the primary focus is on the learners. Have learners in fact mastered the knowledge and skills that the curriculum prescribes? The design of tests to assess learner achievement is a complex subject, as anyone who has written questions for board examinations can amply attest, and it would be helpful for faculty members to better understand some of the issues involved. Deciding how to focus educational assessment can exert major influence on how teachers and learners behave, and spawns a number of interesting questions for educational research. For example, do learners in fact learn the most from the teachers they rate as best?

Another important area of the faculty development curriculum is the use of instructional technology. New learning media, such as Web-based educational materials, open up new possibilities for sharing curricula developing interactive tutorials, tracking learner behavior, and assessing learner comprehension in ways that would have proved nearly impossible in years past. Many faculty members are unfamiliar with the capabilities of the new educational tools of the information age, and this lack of familiarity handicaps our ability to capitalize on them in our teaching. Although there is a limit to how much attention can be devoted to instructional technology in the context of a larger faculty development program, it is important to make faculty members aware of the possibilities, and to provide guidance in how to obtain additional training.

One caveat, however: there is an inevitable tendency for new instructional technologies to so dominate the educational agenda that other crucial aspects of faculty development may be pushed aside. New educational media are only as good as the educators designing them. The quality of the educational product still depends primarily on what and how faculty members are trying to teach, and less on the tools available to do so.

Two final foci of the curriculum of faculty development are presentation skills and communication skills. Presentation skills refer to how faculty put teaching sessions together, including the organization of material, the use of visual aids, and the use of equipment such as laser pointers. Communication skills, by contrast, refer to the nature of the interaction that takes place between teacher and learners. For example, is there in fact a two-way interaction, or is information flowing in one direction only? Does the instructor make effective use of humor and anecdotes, and does the instructor make frequent eye contact? Presentation skills are visible only in the classroom, however, communication skills apply both inside and outside the classroom, including informal teaching opportunities that arise during the workday. Aside from the content of what faculty members are attempting to teach, the quality of our presentation and communication skills can powerfully influence what learners take away from educational interactions.

In designing a curriculum, faculty members should be encouraged to pay close attention to two additional points concerning the alignment of its elements. First, they should attempt to develop a clear and widely shared view of what learners most need to know. A review of the current curriculum often reveals that some of the material being taught is not terribly important. Other material is important, and should be taught wherever time and circumstances permit. Still other material is absolutely critical, and must be taught at all costs. By attempting to differentiate among these different levels of importance, educators can ensure that educational priorities and curricular structure are appropriately aligned.

A second crucial point concerns the different types of curricula that exist in most learning environments. These are the written curriculum, the tested curriculum, and the curriculum that in fact gets taught. It is not infrequent that these three curricula turn out in practice to be very different. For example, a program may have a written curriculum for its residents, but when those stated objectives are compared with what actually gets taught at conferences, the degree of correspondence between the two may turn out to be surprisingly low. Many programs do not know exactly what their residents are being taught, because no one keeps track of it. Moreover, there is often a large gap between what programs say their residents should know and the manner in which they assess learner achievement. Educators should bear in mind that when such gaps exist, learners will usually follow the path prescribed by assessment standards, whether they represent the more important material or not.

What methods work best for faculty development? Given the time constraints in academic medicine, it is tempting to set aside an afternoon or a day for faculty development, based on the presumption that even a short amount of time is better than nothing at all. For example, an outside educational consultant with a background in faculty development might be brought in to give several lectures on how to teach more effectively. In fact, however, 1-day workshops where people are simply told what they ought to be doing usually produce few enduring results. Ongoing sustained programs, in which faculty have the opportunity to revisit teaching on multiple occasions, work best.

The instructors in a faculty development program must understand the knowledge set and practice domains of the faculty. If faculty members are to realize significant improvements in our educational effectiveness, the faculty development curriculum must be grounded in the subject they are in fact teaching. Although many of the principles may be similar, the program used by the local public school system is unlikely to work well for medical school faculty members. Case studies and illustrations should be grounded in the environments in which physicians actually teach. Many faculty members will rapidly tune out an instructor if we think they do not understand what we do.

A variety of faculty development formats might be employed. For example, there is no question that traditional lectures have some role to play. When it comes to providing a basic background in such subjects as learning theory, presentation skills, and educational assessment, good lecturers foster substantial learning in a relatively short period of time. Basing the entire program on lectures, however, is another matter, and would rapidly prove counterproductive. Instead, occasional lectures might be interspersed throughout the program, with other more interactive formats in between. For example, after a lecture on learning theory, faculty members might participate in small group exercises in which they attempt to identify their own preferred approaches to learning.

As noted above, another small group technique that invites active participation is problem-based learning. Groups might read vignettes on different teaching styles, and be asked to provide constructive critiques for improvement. Similarly, videotapes could be used, again asking participants to assess what teachers are doing well, what they are doing poorly, and what suggestions they would make for improvement. Participants could be invited to look at videotapes of their own teaching, as well, or critique one another's teaching styles, with the help of an educational "coach." The goal of such sessions is not only to get participants actively involved in the pursuit of better teaching, but to help them become more self-critical. If people are to improve at anything, they need to recognize first that they could be doing a better job, and second to develop some specific steps they could take to bring about improvement.

Criticism is important, but so is praise. One of the greatest deficiencies in medical education is the dearth of appreciation for teaching. Department chairs and hospital administrators track clinical productivity and research productivity very closely, but teaching is tracked poorly, if at all. As a result, many faculty members simply do not know how well we are doing as educators. Through ongoing faculty development programs, departments can begin to support and foster the faculty's teaching efforts by providing some praise and encouragement. Teaching awards can certainly play a useful role in this process, although those who do not receive awards may soon suppose that they are not very good teachers, and become discouraged.

Another important method of faculty development is to encourage the faculty to become involved in research on teaching. Many aspects of medical education have never been subjected to close scrutiny, and we continue doing them not because we know they work, but because it never occurred to us that there might be a better way of doing things. Consider, for example, the possibility that the quality of medical education might be substantially improved by asking residents to do some writing. Every resident might be asked to write a one-page critique at the end of each rotation, focusing on some aspect of that educational experience that could be improved. Similarly, residents might be asked to write an essay of several pages, each quarter, on topics such as "The Subspecialty That Appeals Most to Me, and Why," or "The Greatest Threat to the Future of My Field." Would residents who participated in such educational activities emerge as better physicians from the 4 years of training? Only through educational research will we ever know.

The faculty should be encouraged to discuss the importance of teaching in the overall mission of the organization. Is excellence in education truly a mission for this group, and what resources is the organization prepared to commit to make it possible? Is teaching sufficiently important that it should play an even more prominent role in departmental decisions on such issues as tenure and promotion? The more teaching excellence represents an important factor in the overall equation of academic success, the more likely are faculty members to devote serious time and attention to the quality of our own teaching. If the faculty agrees that the profile of teaching should be elevated, the introduction of teaching inventories and teaching dossiers can prove to be of great value. Inventories and dossiers encourage faculty to keep a record of instructional activities, teaching development activities, and evidence of teaching quality. Scores on standard evaluation forms are important, but so are anecdotal reports, such as unsolicited letters from students and peers reflecting educational dedication and excellence.

As in other arts in life, learning to teach involves a significant amount of emulation. Discussing theory and participating in group exercises can only take faculty members so far. Ultimately, there is no substitute for exposure to great teachers, and a good faculty development program will involve opportunities to see great teachers at work. In an age when new medical information is readily available through journals and the Internet, continuing to use opportunities to bring in outside speakers, such as visiting professorships, merely to disseminate information makes less and less sense. Instead, some of these resources could be used to establish ongoing workshops in educational best practices, in which master teachers could be shared between institutions to improve educational quality for all. Likewise, other faculty development resources, such as curricula and methods, could be pooled. If departments can collaborate in order to improve the quality of research, why should not education benefit from collaboration as well?

Medical educators must be prepared to make the case that providing a first-rate education for medical students and residents lies in the best interests of their departments and institutions. Rationales for this position would include utilitarian arguments that enhanced education can improve patient care outcomes and lower healthcare costs, as well as professional arguments that teaching is a core activity of medicine, and deserves to be done well. There is no point in undertaking a faculty development program if the institution lacks the resolve to do it right, including a serious commitment of time and money. Merely paying lip service to education can backfire, producing even greater disenchantment among educators.

It would be foolish for an academic healthcare institution to assume that it could provide excellent clinical care or produce first-rate research without making significant capital investments in equipment and supplies. It would be equally foolish for an institution to suppose that it could provide an excellent education without making significant investments in the human capital of its educators. Improving the quality of education is one of the best investments any institution can make, whose "spill-over" benefits in reputation, morale, and ability strengthen everything else it does. Moreover, teaching well is one of the most intrinsically rewarding aspects of being a good physician.

Lessons of Failure

When physicist Paul Lauterbur submitted his first paper to *Nature* concerning what we now call MRI, demonstrating that an imaging technique could, for the first time, differentiate between ordinary water and heavy water, the editors rejected the manuscript, saying among other things that the images were "too fuzzy." Lauterbur rejected their rejection, however, and insisted that they take another look. After further review, they decided to publish the paper, which is now recognized as a classic. Lauterbur later said of the initial rejection, "You could write the entire history of science over the last half century in terms of papers rejected by *Science* or *Nature*."

Error, mistakes, and failure are neither new nor remarkable. What is remarkable is the high degree of intolerance many physicians develop toward failure. Of course, no one sets out to fail. This being said, however, our failure to properly understand and respond to failure is one of the greatest weaknesses of contemporary medicine and biomedical science. Until we learn to regard failure rightly, and educate future physicians to do the same, we are proceeding with eyes half closed. If clinical medicine and biomedical science are to realize their full promise, it is vital that many of us take crash courses in the subject and develop an artist's eye for both the value and the beauty of failure.

Our problem is that we train ourselves in what to do, but we do not educate ourselves in how to learn from what we do. Charles Duell, Commissioner of the US Office of Patents in 1899, is often misquoted as saying, "Everything that can be invented has been invented." If that were true, then there would be no need to go on learning. If not, however, and if, even after more than a century of progress the domain of potential discoveries and inventions still vastly outweighs what we know, then skepticism, curiosity, and creativity are no less important today than at any preceding point in human history.

What is a failure? In simplest terms, a failure might be defined as an event that did not turn out as we intended. Yet if this is the case, failure cannot be an unequivocal misfortune, because it is precisely when the result is different from what we expect that we stand to learn the most. To suppose that everything should turn out exactly as we intend would be the height of hubris, supposing that we had somehow rendered the world itself fully subject to our own ken and control. In fact, however, the world around and within us is too big and complex for us ever to know fully, much less to predict with unerring accuracy, much less still completely to command.

Just as it is possible to succeed well or badly, it is possible to fail badly or well. And in many cases, it is failure that proves most pregnant. In the words of Montaigne, "There are defeats that turn out to be more triumphant than victories." If our objective is to learn, then failure represents an immense opportunity, and if our aim is to seize the greatest opportunities available to us, then we need to become connoisseurs of failure. What constitutes a propitious failure? It is often a project undertaken in pursuit of a noble goal, engaging our best powers, and carried out with both an experimental attitude and a sense of excitement. Above all, it is one we learn from.

Of course, saying that some failures turn out to be blessings begs an important question. From whose point of view are we assessing the balance of benefit over harm? From the standpoint of the educator, scientist, or clinician performing the trial? Or from the perspective of the department, the profession, or society as a whole? One man's meat can be another man's poison. This is precisely what the great physician–writer Chekhov had in mind when he wrote, "One must be a god to be able to tell failures from successes without making a mistake" (Fig. 5.2). The law of unintended consequences can turn out to be as much of a blessing as a curse, and a key task of leadership is to limit the damage of trying out new ideas while enhancing benefits we cannot foresee.

The greater pitfall in the pursuit of knowledge today is not recklessness but excessive caution. For example, the selection processes of many funding organizations are remarkably conservative, encouraging investigators to be predictable

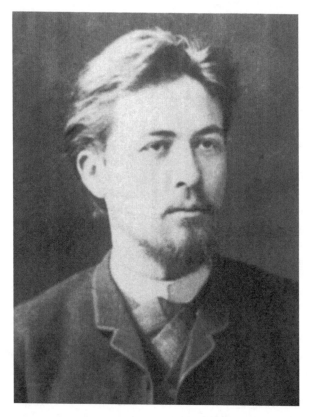

Fig. 5.2 Anton Pavlovich Chekhov (1860–1904). A Russian physician who is also recognized as one of the world's great short story writers. As a student, Chekhov was held back a year at the age of 15 because he failed a Greek exam. Yet he persevered, helping to support his family and paying for his own education by private tutoring and selling short sketches to newspapers. Chekhov once declared, "Medicine is my lawful wife and literature is my mistress." He also insisted that the writer's calling is not to answer questions, but to raise them (Courtesy of Wikimedia Commons)

and safe to the point of seeking funding only for work, the outcome of which they already know. Such systems of funding often do a better job of keeping established investigators funded than promoting the daring pursuit of novel and adventurous lines of inquiry. Fortunately, this danger can be mitigated to some degree by systems of scientific reward that operate retrospectively, such as prizes.

One of the greatest human curses is to get precisely what we want. Consider Ovid's parable of King Midas, who loves wealth so much that he wishes everything he touches would turn into gold. His wish granted, Midas soon realizes to his horror that the fulfillment of his wish represents a terrible curse. We should pray less that our wishes be granted than for the wisdom truly to understand what we aim to do, how we go about it, and how to appraise what we have done. Donald Schön and others have emphasized the importance of reflective practice, whereby we examine not only our results but the models by which we produce them.

This was the genius of Socrates. Instead of merely asking how something could be accomplished as effectively and efficiently as possible, Socrates inquires into the very mental models by which we act. In Plato's dialogues, he is forever urging that we attempt to articulate and examine our objectives and the standards by which we assess success in promoting them. What is truly good, beautiful, and just? What is truly worth knowing? It does not matter how effectively we manage to keep the trains running on time if they are carrying the wrong people to the wrong places. Such a Socratic spirit is never at work when we focus all our energy on merely avoiding failure.

6

Educational Technique

I am not arguing against using computers in school. I am arguing against our sleep-walking attitudes towards it, against allowing it to distract us from important things, against making a god of it.

Neil Postman, *The End of Education*

Assistive Technologies

New educational technologies offer great promise in improving medical education. We should, however, temper our technological enthusiasm with a dose of realism, never forgetting that new technologies cannot outperform the educators who design and implement them. No matter how fancy the bells and whistles, a bad lecture will remain a bad lecture whether it is delivered live or electronically. Uninspired questions will never spark learner curiosity, no matter how dramatic the special effects used to enliven them on a computer screen. While doing our best to make the most of the opportunities new educational technologies afford us, we cannot afford to lose sight of the human side of education.

There are many advantages of new educational technologies, most of which are grounded one way or another in the information technology boom. Information technology provides us with new ways to store, analyze, and convey large amounts of information at very high speeds. This enables learners to access educational material from virtually any site that has a computer and an Internet connection. Moreover, material can be accessed at virtually any time of the day or night. Learners can also spend as much or as little time as they choose with the material, and return to it as many times as they like. Compared to the cost of transporting learners to a central classroom, this also helps reduce costs. In other words, new educational technologies have the potential both to empower and liberate learners. Of course, this is not a new dimension in pedagogy. After all, the introduction of textbooks offered similar benefits, because they too can be studied anywhere at any time and do not require learners or educators to travel to a common meeting place. These are important benefits of new educational technologies, but they are not unique, and thus do not represent a difference in kind from current educational capabilities.

Other strengths of new educational technologies do not duplicate those of printed materials such as textbooks. For example, new educational technologies

R.B. Gunderman, *Achieving Excellence in Medical Education*,
DOI: 10.1007/978-0-85729-307-7_6, © Springer-Verlag London Limited 2011

make it possible to integrate text, images, and sounds in ways that standard textbooks cannot. This offers immense advantages in teaching medical students how to interpret chest radiographs or recognize different heart sounds. They can also access and organize educational materials for themselves, in an individualized fashion, in ways that extend beyond flipping through a textbook or journal. For example, some learners may prefer an educational approach focused on graphics, and others may prefer a text-based approach. Both can be offered to learners, who then customize the material to their own learning preferences.

An even greater benefit of the new educational technologies is the greater degree of interaction they permit. Material can be presented in a question-and-answer format that helps learners evaluate their performance and identify their own strengths and weaknesses. An interactive approach to software design can enable learners to play a more active role in their own education, so that they are not merely absorbing information as they read. For example, learners can be challenged to use what they are learning to solve problems. If they succeed, they can be offered new material and new problems to solve. If they fail to demonstrate an adequate grasp of the material, they can be offered remedial content. This interactive component can make learning more enjoyable as well, because learners are actively engaged in putting the material to use.

Educational technology can also permit more frequent and timely revision of educational materials. For example, text can be updated and revised as the need arises. There is no need to wait until several years have passed to issue another edition, or wait to accumulate a sufficient number of new findings to justify the publication of an entirely new article. This ensures that learners are able to concentrate on the most up-to-date material, and suggestions for improvement, including those offered by learners themselves, can be immediately capitalized upon. Likewise, obsolete material can be immediately deleted, whereas with printed material there is always a danger that some learner may be misled by it until the book or journal article is destroyed.

New educational technologies can also provide educators with valuable insights into how learners are using the material, which can be used to enhance our educational programs. Such information can be difficult and costly to provide to authors of conventional textbooks and journal articles. When are learners accessing the material? How long do they spend with it, and how often do they return to it? How do they order their progression through it? Which portions are they skipping entirely? How much time do they spend working with images and diagrams, how much time on the text, and how much time on self-assessment questions? How do they rate various sections, and what suggestions for improvement can they share?

If learners are taking self-assessment tests as they move through the material, how well are they performing? Where do they seem to master the material with ease? With which questions do they have the most difficulty? Can we predict, based on educational background, where particular learners are likely to encounter the most difficulties, and tailor their instruction accordingly? Where opportunities for improvement emerge, the educational approach can be altered to facilitate learning effectiveness.

The so-called hypermedia and simulation devices can assess not only cognitive performance, but skills acquisition, as well. Learners can perform their first procedures on real patients after having acquired considerably more practice, thereby reducing learner anxiety and enhancing patient comfort and safety. This may also lower the cost of education by reducing reliance on expensive laboratory animals on which learners can practice.

Despite its many advantages, however, new educational technology is not an entirely unmixed blessing, and we need to be as cognizant of its limitations as we are of its benefits. One such limitation is the evidence supporting their increased efficiency and effectiveness. Can we say with confidence that new educational technologies produce the same level of proficiency with a decreased investment of educator time, money, and effort? Will they, for example, enable us to expend fewer hours each week of faculty time on education, because learners are now devoting more time to computer-based interactive learning? Given the increased pressure on the time of faculty members, this could be important. New technologies that make it possible to reduce faculty teaching commitments could become very attractive.

We also need to better understand the effect of new educational technologies on educational effectiveness. Enhanced efficiency means we can achieve the same results at lower cost. Enhanced effectiveness means we can achieve better results. Perhaps new educational technologies produce higher scores on standard tests. To adequately assess some of the most novel aspects of new educational technologies, it is likely that new forms of testing will need to be devised.

Yet educational technology is not a panacea. We cannot solve the educational problems that face us merely by investing more heavily in new educational technology, any more than we can improve our commute to work by investing in a new automobile (Fig. 6.1). We cannot simply substitute computers and interactive software for lecturers, and rest assured that we will be better off. Many empirical studies of new educational technologies demonstrate no substantial difference in learner performance compared to more traditional modes of learning, and in other cases experimental design is so confounded that no clear inferences can be drawn. This is not to suggest that we should give up on testing new educational technologies. Instead we need to redouble our efforts to perform rigorous tests. We should not, however, lapse into the assumption that something new, sophisticated, or expensive is necessarily better.

In many cases, new educational technology can be shown to be superior. However, it is often the improved quality of the curriculum or another aspect of educational design, rather than the technology itself, that is responsible for the improvement. As we have seen, the dross of a mediocre or poor curriculum cannot be turned into educational gold merely by adding the catalyst of a computer. We also need to keep careful track of the development costs of such educational technologies. In some cases, the investment of faculty and support staff time may be so great that the reduction in face-to-face contact time is more than offset. Designing high-quality materials using the latest educational technology is no less demanding than writing a textbook.

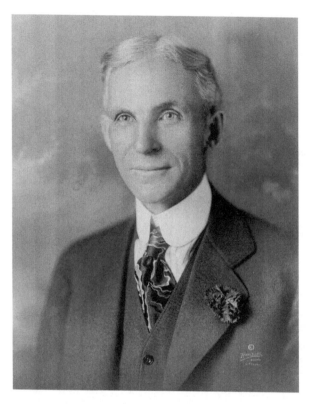

Fig. 6.1 Henry Ford (1863–1947). Founder of the Ford Motor Company and inventor of the Model T, which brought automobiles to ordinary Americans, Ford promulgated the assembly line technique of mass production, dramatically increasing productivity and lowering costs. Ford wrote, "I will build a car for the great multitude. It will be large enough for the family, but small enough for the individual to run and care for. It will be constructed of the best materials, by the best men to be hired, after the simplest designs that modern engineering can devise. But it will be so low in price that no man making a good salary will be unable to own one—and enjoy with his family the blessing of hours of pleasure in God's great open spaces." In what respects are Ford's techniques of mass production an appropriate model for medical education, and where might such an approach lead us astray? (Courtesy of Wikimedia Commons)

One of the most important confounding variables in the assessment of new educational technologies is the enthusiasm of their proponents. We must be careful to ensure that we do not adopt evaluation rubrics inherently biased in favor of new technologies. Interactive computer-based tutorials may be excellent at fostering learning in some areas, such as conveying basic principles, but not so effective in other areas, such as the development of interpersonal skills. We have a tendency to invest more time and effort in new innovations for which we are responsible. This can bias investigation toward new technologies, because the people responsible for them make no comparable investment in time and energy in improving traditional educational materials.

Regardless of how effective a new educational technology turns out to be, we should never expect that face-to-face interaction between learners and educators will be entirely supplanted. Many important lessons about excelling as a physician can only be learned in actual practice, through a variation on the apprenticeship model. How do we learn how to interact with patients? By watching and working with people who already know how to do it. Is there only one right way of doing so? Often there is not, and it is important that we respect the diversity of practice styles in the way we educate the next generation of physicians. Certainly, some approaches are simply wrong, and some are more effective than others, but lessons such as work ethic and responses to failure probably cannot be taught any other way. These lessons could never be conveyed very well by textbooks, and they probably cannot be conveyed well by computers either.

It is also unlikely, at least for the foreseeable future, that computer software can outperform real educators at responding to learner questions. Doing so requires a high level of understanding, responsiveness, and genuine concern with the well-being of learners that no computer can replicate. We can include responses to frequently asked questions in the software, but it is unlikely that we can anticipate every good question. We aim not merely to transmit information, but to enhance the curiosity and incisiveness of learners, and this requires that we encourage learners to pose new questions and make ourselves available to help answer them.

We must also guard against the potentially deleterious effects of technologies that seek to replace the live educator. This may remove much of the enticement to teach, and may deprive some of our best and most dedicated educators of one of the greatest rewards of teaching, namely, the opportunity to interact in real time with learners. There is no question that every educator eventually reaches a point of diminishing marginal returns, where additional hours of learner contact time merely reduce their educational effectiveness. If the demands are too great, educators may burn out. Yet somewhere below that threshold lies an important level of educational commitment that many of us need in order to remain excited about medical education. We need to look into the eyes of learners, and to converse with them face-to-face, to know what effect we are having.

The single learner hunkered down over a computer offers a number of advantages as a model for education, but it also manifests some weaknesses. It is equally important that learners enjoy an opportunity to learn together in one another's company. If learning is in part a social activity involving the shared construction of understanding, then learners need to work together, and we need to provide opportunities to share perspectives, collaborate, and form friendships. Learners relying strictly on computer-based distance education will be deprived of such opportunities.

Above all, we must guard against the temptation to allow our fascination with new technologies to drive our educational vision. Educational technology is not an end in itself, but a means to an end. Consider a culinary analogy. We could base our menu on the food preparation devices we have available in the kitchen, or we could base it on the exigencies of human nutrition and the preferences of the human palate. Both are important, but there is clearly something wrong with a kitchen that bases all decisions on what to serve strictly on its equipment. Perhaps we need to get some new equipment, or perhaps we need to get rid of some we have. How do we know? Based on what we like and need to eat. The same goes for education. We need to understand what students most need to know, and use our educational technology accordingly.

Minds and Machines

In the 1970s, it would have been difficult to conceive the effects new developments in information technology would have on education. Who could have imagined that many learners would be able to carry around personal computers no bulkier than a book, that whole medical charts could be reduced to the size of a personal digital assistant and connected directly with hospital information systems, and that new software would make it possible for learners to interact directly with images and text, without the mediating presence of a live instructor, or that an electronic network called the World Wide Web would permit the nearly instantaneous dissemination of educational materials at incredibly low cost? Just beyond the horizon lie technologies that superimpose networks of information onto our daily lives and provide just-in-time access to databases and decision support resources.

Some uses of educational technology may be regarded as traditional, such as placing the content of a book or journal article online. Others, such as interactive software, are more innovative, and still others, such as simulation devices, may prove to be truly revolutionary. At one time, such technologies as the carousel slide projector, the calculator, photocopier, the slide rule, and the printing press were regarded as radical innovations. As new technologies continue to open up new possibilities for sharing knowledge, they will continue to shape medical education. We should welcome those that help us meet our core educational missions by increasing the effectiveness and efficiency of learning. To understand when we are really realizing such benefits, however, we need to be mindful of certain fundamental concepts of human learning that provide the foundation for incorporating new educational technologies into medical education. Three such concepts are the three distinct cognitive levels of medicine: information, knowledge, and understanding. Depending on which of these three cognitive levels we seek to address, the potential roles of new educational technologies will differ.

Information is the level of facts or data. When we convey information, we simply transfer it from one location to another, just as we might download a file from the Internet to the hard drive of a computer. Medicine is chock full of such information, including laboratory results, lists of differential diagnoses, and the risk factors for particular disease processes. When we think of sharing information, we think in terms of a transmission model of education. The goal of the educator is to move information into students from some outside source, such as the words the educator is speaking or the information contained in a particular reading assignment. Transferring information requires relatively little effort on the part of the educator, at least to the extent that the information contained in a lecture might be transmitted equally effectively by a recording, which would not require the educator to be present.

One of the drawbacks of a strictly informational account of medical education is the fact that information transferred often lacks context and purpose. And when ideas lack context and purpose, they often remain relatively inert in the mind of the learner. For example, the information might be recalled and recited when the learner is appropriately prompted, but otherwise it might not be available for day-to-day problem solving. I may be able to recite the information on cardiopulmonary resuscitation contained on the instruction card in my wallet, yet be utterly incapable of applying that information effectively in a real-life emergency.

Another drawback of information is the ease with which it can inundate us like a flood, so that learners soon feel that we are drowning in it. The ability of new information technologies to transmit information more easily, more quickly, and less expensively means that the risk of information overload is becoming progressively more acute. We soon lose our bearings, and do not know how new information fits together with other concepts within and between domains. When that happens, new information may be essentially meaningless. Thus we cannot assume that more time in the classroom, longer and more extensive reading assignments, and greater educator effort necessarily translate into improved learning outcomes. In some cases, adopting such seemingly desirable policies may in fact prove counterproductive, resulting in reduced learner performance. For these reasons, it is impossible to achieve mastery or even competency in any field operating strictly at the level of information.

Knowledge may be conceptualized as information with a purpose. In the educational context, knowledge sharing involves both a sender and receiver, but it implies that at least the sender, and ideally the receiver as well, aim to foster the development of some new understanding or capability in the learner. As a result of the sharing of the knowledge, the learner should be changed in some way that shows up in behavior, ideas, or perspectives. Perhaps the learner understands the medical meaning of the term inflammation, begins to develop skill at placing an intravenous catheter, or grasps for the first time what it is like to look up at a group of physicians from a hospital bed. Knowledge is more likely than information to be retained and understood by the learner simply because it implies an intention on the part of the educator to impart something or on the part of the learner to understand something.

An example of knowledge is the material discussed in a traditional didactic lecture, where the lecturer has attempted to get across to the learners some theme or series of concepts. If the model of learning is strictly one way, then we are still talking about a kind of transmission, in which learners operate in a primarily passive, receptive mode. Yet it is not the same as mere information transfer, in the sense that the educator is trying to make the material meaningful to the learners.

Regarding technology, there is a risk that we become so enamored of our new devices that we forget our educational mission. Collecting information and putting it together in new ways is not, by itself, a recipe for enhanced understanding.

We need to link knowledge to learners' prior experience. If we are teaching medical students how to recognize a particular physical examination finding, such as clubbing of the digits, we need to offer them insight into why clubbing is important and what could be causing it. We could never fail to recognize a case of clubbing, but if we do not know how to put that insight to use in the care of the patient, then its clinical utility is limited at best. On the other hand, if learners understand why clubbing is important, then we will be in a better position to study it in the first place.

The transferability of inert knowledge is poor, but dynamic knowledge can be transferred from one situation to another, because it has been thoroughly integrated into the learner's experience. We need to be able to see how what we are learning fits into a larger context, so that we can draw relevant distinctions, recognize relevant connections, and situate what we know in its most useful context. We might think of prior knowledge as a kind of scaffolding or framework into which new knowledge needs to be fitted. The more niches that scaffolding offers, the more likely we are to be able to find a place or places in which to situate it. For example, to be useful, we must connect knowledge to our understanding of the circumstances in which it applies. This is why hands-on simulation exercises are such a crucial part of training in cardiopulmonary resuscitation.

Like information, knowledge has limitations. For example, it does not tell us what it should be used for, nor does it show us how different knowledge domains fit together. It also leaves us unsure about what is most worth knowing. Again, we can pour more and more knowledge onto the heads of learners, but that alone will not improve their preparation to learn on their own. Learners need, more than merely, to know a lot, we also need to be able to discern what is more or less important to learn, and to be able to direct our own learning of it. This is where understanding comes in. When we really understand a topic or a domain, we grasp what is most worth knowing about it, and how it fits together with other domains of our knowledge. When we study medicine, we face a seemingly insurmountable challenge, namely, the fact that we cannot know as much as there is to know. We must make choices, or someone else must make them for us, about what is most worth knowing. We need to prioritize our learning. To do this, we need to know how that knowledge will be useful during our practice. We also need to know what aspects of a subject we need to know "cold," and which we merely need to know well enough to be able to look them up in a reference work.

Someone who not only knows but understands medicine understands its fundamental characteristics, the domains of knowledge that are most essential to it, how such knowledge can be put to use for the benefit of patients, what questions are most worth investigating about it, and perhaps even something about how to learn it and therefore teach it. Generally speaking, it takes years, perhaps even decades, to develop deep understanding of a complex domain such as medicine, but there are strategies we can pursue as educators to try to make the learning process as effective and efficient as possible. For example, if learners are studying a particular medical discipline, we can encourage them to try to understand the role that that discipline plays in the larger scheme of healthcare, where its practitioners can make the greatest contributions to patients, and what conditions need to be in place for that potential to be realized.

Information can be conveyed through transmission and knowledge can be conveyed through statements, but understanding is fostered largely through questioning. This is one of the great insights embodied in the so-called Socratic Method, which seeks to draw out understanding through questioning. If we are going to understand something, we need to become actively engaged in reflecting on it, attempting to discover for ourselves what it means and why it is important. Socrates' method of interacting with his interlocutors was not so much to tell them things as to stimulate them by questioning to think for themselves. It is simply impossible to acquire genuine understanding in a passive fashion. The learner must be an active inquirer, or at least coinvestigator, with the educator.

The challenge of using educational technology to facilitate learning increases as we move up the scale from information to knowledge to understanding. It is very easy to use an electronic network to transfer a large load of information to a learner. It is considerably more difficult to foster real understanding without face-to-face interactions between educators and learners. We make a grave mistake if we suppose that educational technology alone can somehow receive information and organize and convey it to learners in a way that makes it memorable, usable, and valuable in creating a deep sense of the cognitive domain of medicine. To move from novice to expert requires an enormous amount of instruction, practice, and reflection by both learners and educators. New educational technologies can make many learning tasks more efficient and even more effective. It can present content in ways that learners find congenial. However, it cannot substitute for an enlightened educator.

We cannot simply strap our old educational content onto new electronic media and expect them to boost our educational effectiveness into the stratosphere, because electronic media such as the Internet are equally good at delivering very good and very poor materials. New educational technologies can no more transform learning than buying a new truck could change the nutritional value of the groceries we deliver. Studies demonstrating that new educational technologies can enhance learning outcomes are so commonplace that they now often generate little interest. The educational effectiveness, however, often has less to do with the technology itself than with the instructional design. Poorly designed programs will not enhance learning no matter how sophisticated the technology that delivers them. Technology inappropriately applied will actually degrade, not enhance, our educational outcomes.

We must not forget that knowledge and especially understanding are shared in communities, where learning is like acquiring a new language. To excel as physicians, we need not only to retain a large collection of facts, but to act as excellent physicians act. This has to do with habits of practice, and with matters of character, as much as with cognition. A great deal of what we know, which Michael Polanyi called tacit knowledge, cannot be written down. We must work side by side, and converse with one another about what we are doing. These are learning objectives that an isolated learner perched in front of a computer screen may never be able to realize.

Quality

One of the most important challenges in educating future health professionals is to help them develop a sense of quality, and the means by which we assess quality represents a vital educational technology. Can we reliably and accurately differentiate between mediocre and great physicians? What would we need to know about a physician or a medical practice to determine whether or not it is great? Would the volume of patients tell the tale? How about the number of procedures or amount of revenue generated? What about error rates, or conformity with recommended pathways? How about patient satisfaction scores? Would we need to know something about health outcomes? Could we identify great physicians from medical records, or would we need to observe them in action to discern greatness?

Seven key constituents of quality are precision, accuracy, safety, efficiency, efficacy, value, and appropriateness. Precision refers to how tightly results are clustered together, the reproducibility of findings. Do different physicians looking at the same patient reach the same conclusions regarding whether or not the patient is ill, the number and nature of positive findings, the differential diagnostic possibilities, and the appropriate course of further diagnostic evaluation or treatment? If precision is low, confidence is likely to suffer, yet precision alone is not sufficient to guarantee high-quality medicine. There are still situations where even large numbers of observers may be wrong, for example, the failure of many physicians at a premier medical center to diagnose former US first lady Eleanor Roosevelt's disseminated tuberculosis in time to institute appropriate therapy. This is especially likely in situations where independence of assessment is low or the imperative for consensus is high. The pressure to achieve consensus may outweigh the need to reach the correct conclusion.

In contrast to precision, which refers to variability, accuracy concerns the degree to which impressions correctly represent reality. Pathology has often been regarded as the final arbiter of truth, but this is not always justified. Pathologists are fallible, and sometimes make mistakes. Aside from the difficulty of establishing "gold standards" against which to assay medical conclusions is another important limitation on the assessment of accuracy. In many cases, conclusions are never subjected to rigorous verification. For example, we treat many infections empirically, without ever isolating the responsible organism. The patient gets better, and we do not know for sure whether the therapy was responsible for the improvement. The point is not that medicine is inherently unreliable, but simply that many diagnoses remain hypotheses, and should be treated as such.

Since the era of Hippocrates, one of the first principles of medicine has been, "Do no harm." The concept of safety is represented by the ethical principle of nonmaleficence, which states that health professionals should protect patients from harm. Of course, safety is not quite so simple. For one thing, there is the issue of whose safety the physician is called upon to look out for. Does the umbrella of professional responsibility extend only to patients under the physician's direct care, or to other patients, family members, health professionals and other employees of the healthcare organization, and the community at large? In some cases, safety may be legitimately compromised for the sake of innovation. Preventing investigators and patients from taking risks to which reasonable people might reasonably agree in order to advance knowledge and improve current standards of diagnosis and therapy would be a mistake.

Efficiency may be defined as the ratio of results achieved to resources expended. Such resources may include time, effort, and money. In an era where commerce plays an increasing role in healthcare, there is a strong tendency to focus on fungible resources, those that can be valued in dollars and cents. Yet wise physicians know that the job most worth having is not necessarily the one that pays the most. The steps necessary to maximize the economic efficiency of a medical practice might entail the neglect of other goals that make physicians' work meaningful and rewarding. At some point, increases in productivity may require substantial reductions in quality of work life, with increased rates of burnout, errors, and defections, and associated losses in morale and fulfillment. A relentless focus on efficiency, and in particular, on one aspect of efficiency, can ultimately undermine the performance and produce more harm than benefit.

Efficacy focuses on the relative effectiveness of alternative courses of action, disregarding the risks and costs of each. Efficacy is highly desirable, but needs to be tempered by other considerations, including efficiency. For example, we could dramatically decrease the incidence of cancer in various organs such as the thyroid gland, the breast, and the gonads, by surgically removing them. The efficacy of this practice, measured in terms of the reduction in risk of cancer, would be very high. Yet the simple fact that an intervention has a high level of efficacy does not reliably establish it as the appropriate alternative, and the pursuit of quality has its limits. In some situations, a product, service, or performance of lower quality is not only acceptable but actually preferable. For example, most of us would prefer to hear "Happy Birthday" sung by our own friends and loved ones than by a world famous vocalist. In musical terms, the quality may be lower, but it means more to us.

This introduces the crucial theme of value. What is value, as opposed to quality? Value concerns the ratio of quality over price or cost. In most circumstances in life, it makes sense to settle for less than the very best, because achieving the absolute highest level of quality is so costly that it quickly displaces other worthy goals. If the clinical situation involves an acute, life-threatening diagnosis that mandates immediate treatment—for example, a patient with suspected aortic dissection—then even the most expensive test may be warranted. In other situations, however, less costly alternatives may be more appropriate. For example, most patients with low back pain will derive little benefit from costly diagnostic tests and back surgery. It is ironic but true that the best is often not in fact the best—that is, the highest technology, most sensitive, and costliest option is not the most appropriate choice for most patients. The issue is not just one of value, but one of appropriateness.

Appropriateness is situational. It depends on the who, what, when, where, how, and why of the situation. To determine an appropriate course of action requires knowledge of the specific circumstances. Is the patient a world-class athlete or a nursing home resident? Is the suspected lesion a disc herniation or a metastasis? Did the symptoms arise in the past few days or have they been present off and on for years? Are we seeing the case in the course of routine clinical practice or consulting on a medicolegal dispute? Is the patient seeking consultation to prove fitness for work or competition or in hopes of receiving compensation for injuries suffered on the job? Depending on the answers to such questions, the appropriate diagnostic recommendations may differ substantially.

In other words, discernment will remain an indispensible and irreducible aspect of high-quality medical practice. It is indispensible because, when it comes to applying general principles to particular situations, there is no substitute for a thorough understanding of the particulars. It is irreducible because no level of detail and sophistication in clinical pathways, algorithms, and heuristics can ever replace the perspective of an expert who knows the distinctive features of the situation well. We want quality, but not at the expense of value. And we want value, but not at the expense of appropriateness. Ultimately, educating great physicians means not only transferring knowledge and skills, but cultivating the faculty of discernment, which manifests itself nowhere more so than in educators' level of respect and trust in their pupils.

There is much to be learned from nonmedical sources, but medicine is a distinct field marked by distinctive quality considerations. What works in manufacture, where the goal may be merely to reduce deviations from a standard, may not work in healthcare, where patients and providers differ from one another in important respects. Every physician has a professional responsibility to pursue improvements in quality, and doing so can be one of the most fulfilling aspects of a career, enriching the care of patients and helping colleagues practice better medicine. Medical educators need to be vigilant, creative, and energetic advocates for quality in the healthcare system. To do so, however, we require a rich understanding of the relationship between quality, value, and appropriateness, so that we focus quality improvement efforts on the most important questions. Doing so requires more than scientific rigor. It requires discernment and artistry.

7

Obstacles to Excellence

Everyone thinks of changing the world, but no one thinks of changing himself.

Leo Tolstoy, *The Kingdom of God Is Within You*

Assessing Outcomes

How do we know whether our educational programs are achieving their goals? Medicine itself has experienced a movement toward outcomes assessment, grounded in the view that we cannot really know whether medicine works if we do not undertake an assessment of outcomes, and this trend has affected medical education, as well. We can say how many hours students spend in the classroom, the curriculum they are expected to study, and how many faculty members are involved in teaching them, but we really need to know what the students are learning and what they are able to do as a result. This has spawned interest in such evaluative techniques as objective structured clinical examinations, where students are asked to demonstrate their ability to take histories and perform physical examinations, rather than merely answer multiple-choice questions.

This growing interest in outcomes assessment is in most respects salutary. Medical education, like medicine itself, cannot afford to proceed in the dark, and the better we understand the results we are achieving, the more effectively we can align our programs with our objectives. However, the assessment of outcomes is not necessarily a benign enterprise. The introduction of new research methodologies, the growth in professional interest, and new funding opportunities do not prove that the effort itself is sound. If we go about it in a misguided fashion, assessing educational outcomes can actually do more harm than good. I know of a secondary school teacher who laments the impact of outcomes assessment on his students. "Oh, how I could teach if only I didn't have to teach to the examinations," the implication being that the national trend toward outcomes assessment has actually "dumbed down" the quality of students' education. If educational outcomes assessment is to realize its full potential, it is vital that it conduct its own ongoing critical self-assessment and reappraisal. We need to be especially clear about the nature of the outcomes we wish to assess, the purposes behind their assessment, and the means by which we evaluate and utilize the information we acquire.

R.B. Gunderman, *Achieving Excellence in Medical Education*,
DOI: 10.1007/978-0-85729-307-7_7, © Springer-Verlag London Limited 2011

Determining the relative efficacy, effectiveness, benefit-to-cost ratio, or cost-effectiveness of any educational program requires that we make some basic assumptions. Under what conditions will the testing be performed? What instruments will be used to collect the data? According to what standards will the data be analyzed? But perhaps most important of all, what are we trying to define, measure, and evaluate? Let us suppose for the moment that medical schools exist to help transform bright college graduates into physicians. Is our primary duty to help each of those students to complete their education? What if some of them turn out not to like medicine, or not to be very good at it? Or is our purpose to meet the healthcare needs of society? If the latter, then what are the implications for affirmative action in admission policies, and how do we balance that mission against the rights of students to be evaluated based on their academic merits?

We might, for example, say that the medical school's mission is to provide an education that optimizes the ratio of education to cost. Yet as soon as we make cost a component of our evaluation, certain aspects of medical education tend to take a back seat, and these are outcomes on which the vitality and integrity of the medical profession, and ultimately the health of patients, powerfully depend. For example, what happens to ethics and our attitude toward knowledge?

Every physician who cares not only for patients but for the profession of medicine has an interest in ensuring that it remains a challenging, enjoyable, and meaningful endeavor. This is especially true of academicians, who play a large role in educating the next generation of physicians. The manner in which we implement educational outcomes assessment will exert a powerful effect on how we view the practice of medicine. Do we, for example, want to retain individual initiative and creativity in medical education, or insofar as possible, define a single educational program that everyone should follow? It may turn out that the engagement of educators in the educational enterprise hinges to an important degree on their own sense of having helped to design the education they are providing. Why should I pour myself into educating medical students when everything I do and say has been prescribed by someone else?

There are problems with conceiving medical education as a business. On the one hand, our educational institutions cannot survive if we ignore sound business practices. Yet, if we begin to view what we do as a business, then the educational mission is likely to suffer. There is a big difference between seeing the medical school as an educational institution that needs sound business advice and seeing it as a business that happens to deliver education as its principal product. Can we, for example, measure the worth of an education in terms of dollars and cents? Certainly, we can describe the value of a Doctor of Medicine degree in lifetime earnings. But can we truly encompass what it means to become a physician, and especially a very good physician, in financial terms? If we cannot translate that transformation from layperson to physician into dollars, then the role of a business mentality will require careful examination.

Do we suppose that the outcomes of medical education are merely an economic outcome? There is no question that knowledge can be considered an element of human capital, a factor in the equation describing the cost of healthcare.

The gradual replacement of physicians by businesspeople as the leaders of our hospitals and healthcare organizations indicates that such a transition is already well underway. Community hospitals and even medical schools have been assimilated by healthcare corporations. It no longer sounds strange to hear patients referred to as healthcare consumers, or even customers. Yet, what is our model of the patient–physician relationship? Should it be one dominated by the motto of the marketplace: *caveat emptor,* buyer beware? Or should it be one characterized above all by mutual respect and trust? If, in the name of improving the bottom lines of our medical schools, we begin to regard the patient–physician relationship and the learner–educator relationship as a mere market transaction, then the bottom line, the lowest common economic denominator, will soon rule. Medical education will finally become the business that some health economists have long argued it should be.

Yet even such seemingly objective educational outcomes as costs and benefits and cost-effectiveness are in fact relative terms. They are always, at least implicitly, relative to the cost of some other option, or even the cost of doing nothing. Objective answers and quantified data are not always merely true or complete, because the type of question we pose influences the substance of the answer we receive. It is no surprise that when we ask a businessperson a question, we receive an economic answer. But before we pose such a question, we should satisfy ourselves that the businessperson is the right person to query. And this is a question we must answer without business guidance. Do we envision a future of medical education in which businesspeople largely define and control what counts as medical education's product, how it is delivered, and at what cost? How we understand educational outcomes assessment will have a huge impact on its ethical outcomes. If we implement it as a means to enable dedicated medical educators to do a better job of educating the next generation of physicians, then its effect may be quite salutary. On the other hand, its effect may prove quite deleterious if we conceive of it primarily as a means to subjugate an unruly faculty and force them to practice a less expensive form of medical education.

Educational outcomes assessment invites us to inspect our medical epistemology, and reexamine perennial questions that lie at its heart. What do we know? What counts as medical knowledge? If there is a single factor that explains the tremendous explosion in biomedical knowledge in the past century, it is the application of a new scientific method to health and disease. If we begin thinking strictly in terms of educational outcomes, we may undermine this framework, supplanting cause-and-effect reasoning with reliance on probabilities. Statistical associations leave out a crucial scientific question: Why? We must cultivate a curiosity about underlying causes of success and failure, one that strict reliance on outcomes might easily erode.

Nor do we want to do away with the personal experiences of medical educators. The great medical educator is as much an artist as a scientist, able to apply broad principles to particular learners and situations. This requires the development of insight and a wealth of personal experience. There is no recipe in a cookbook for a master educator. What works in many cases will not necessarily

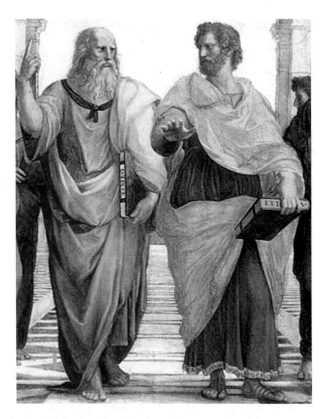

Fig. 7.1 Detail of Raphael's *The School of Athens*, depicting Plato (*left*, 428–348 BC) and Aristotle (384–322 BC). Both philosophers argued that knowledge is important not only because it may prove useful, but also for its own sake. In fact, Aristotle opens his most essential work, *Metaphysics*, with the statement, "All human beings naturally desire to know." Are such medical disciplines as anatomy, physiology, pathology, diagnosis, and therapy worth knowing merely because they are useful in caring for patients, or is such knowledge at least partly choice worthy for its own sake? (Courtesy of Wikimedia Commons)

work in every case, and sometimes the difference between a merely good educator and a great educator is the ability to spot the distinctive features of a particular educational situation. Nor do we want to be in the position of asserting that the value of knowledge is purely utilitarian. Knowing is in itself a worthy end of medicine (Fig. 7.1).

The discovery and sharing of knowledge are also intrinsically worthy objectives. Measurement of educational outcomes tends to be tied to the present, or more accurately, the recent past. We cannot always assess the value of knowledge or the probability of acquiring it in prospective terms. We simply do not know where every investigation will lead. The return on investment might take years or even decades or more to calculate, and even then, we may not truly understand which investigations contributed to the final result. The textbooks of today are terribly useful, but they cannot tell us what should be in the textbooks of tomorrow. Likewise, we cannot always predict which investments of faculty time and energy will pay the greatest dividends.

Educational outcomes assessment has the potential to enhance our educational performance, but only as long as we clearly understand the outcomes we are trying to achieve, and the limitations of the techniques we employ. Every successful effort to assess educational outcomes must be situated in a larger understanding of the purposes of medical education, and ultimately of medicine itself.

Bullshit

Educators naturally tend to focus a great deal of attention on pressing issues such as budgets, learning space and equipment, and assessment techniques, but one of the most crucial obstacles to educational excellence concerns a more fundamental educational objective: a healthy sense of respect for the truth. Among the most intriguing philosophical books published in the first decade of the new millennium was a slim monograph on this very topic, by Princeton University philosopher Harry Frankfurt. Entitled simply if idiomatically, *On Bullshit* (Princeton University Press, 2005), Frankfurter's work exposes the origins and implications of this sadly pervasive feature of contemporary life. Even the medical profession is not free of it. What can we do to decrease the prevalence of bullshitting among the next generation of physicians?

Frankfurt defines bullshit as deliberate misrepresentation. It is not, however, synonymous with lying. When people tell a lie, they do so intending to mislead. In so doing, they are very mindful of the difference between truth and falsity. Liars recognize what is true and what is false, and attempt to convince the listener that what is false is in fact true. This sort of deception underlies most scientific and literary misconduct, where data have been falsified or writers have attempted to take credit for someone else's work. We know the truth, but we choose to say something else.

Bullshit is different. Though it too is a form of deliberate misrepresentation, bullshitters do not really care whether what they are saying is true or not. Bullshitters merely do not want to be revealed as unknowing. They want everyone to think they know what they are talking about, so even when they do not, they go ahead and act as if they do. They care most about appearances, and they will say what they need to say in order to maintain the impression of authority. To tell a lie, it is necessary to know the truth, but to bullshit it is only necessary not to care about it.

Of course, bullshit is the namesake of excrement. Frankfurt describes excrement as the "corpse" of nourishment, or what remains after the vital elements in food have been exhausted. In this sense, bullshit is an appropriate term for this form of mendacity, because it belies the very essence of communication. Consider the ancient philosophical puzzle called the Epimenides paradox: "Everything I tell you is a lie." Yet how can everything I say be a lie if this very statement, asserting that I lie, is itself a lie? Would this not indicate that I am telling the truth?

Communication is only possible when we can assume a shared system of meaning respected by both parties. Like the boy who cried wolf, if student physicians habitually mislead, they will soon gain the reputation of untrustworthiness. Even when they seek earnestly to tell the truth, they may not be believed. A student, professor, colleague, or friend who has lost the trust of others has suffered one of the most serious professional injuries. Trust is perhaps the most fundamental of all virtues in the professions, where we put allegiance to truth over the promotion of self-interest.

Why is bullshit on the rise? Frankfurt asserts that bullshit is inevitable in situations that require us to talk or write about something that we do not understand, a perpetual hazard for physicians in the increasingly complex world of medicine. This is a danger in perpetuating the myth of the omniscient physician. It promotes in patients, colleagues, and perhaps even ourselves the expectation that there is nothing we do not know. If learners begin to feel that they cannot admit ignorance without harming their grade or destroying their self-image, and therefore feel obliged to make pronouncements on every topic they encounter, they will have joined the ranks of the bullshitters.

When a conversation shifts to a topic about which we know nothing, we face an important choice. We can either remain silent, or at least admit our ignorance, or we can bullshit. The most truthful course of action, of course, is to remain silent, or at least to admit that we do not know. For people whose sense of pride and very self-identity are bound up with knowing, the greater temptation is to speak. Who will be the biggest bullshitters of all? People who feel obliged to render an opinion on everything. Unfortunately, taking on formal authority can augment this impulse, making the temptation even greater for leaders and would-be leaders.

Of course, hiding our ignorance is not the only reason we bullshit. There is also the impulse to avoid unpleasant or threatening aspects of daily life. For example, we may downplay or seek to explain away signs of a brewing storm in a patient's care in an effort to distract others and ourselves from unpleasant prospects. We may fail to broach in a timely fashion important questions surrounding end-of-life care. If we are to avoid this pitfall, we must be willing to look threats in the eye. When someone has something unpleasant to tell us, we must be prepared to give a full hearing rather than escape at the first opportunity. When the time is nigh, we must be prepared to broach the topic ourselves.

Another reason we bullshit is the desire to avoid an otherwise embarrassing silence. Rather than allow a lull in the conversation to go on for more than a few seemingly interminable seconds, someone chimes in with an inapposite point that merely distracts everyone from what really needs to be said. This is a terrible pitfall in the practice of medicine, when patients and colleagues may need a few minutes to compose themselves before they can find the words to say what really needs to be said. In this respect, silence can be golden, for it is sometimes only in silence that the truth can emerge.

Frankfurt suggests that a new bullshit-friendly attitude is exacerbating our contemporary situation. This is the view, not unknown among medical students and residents, that there is no objective reality, no truth with a capital T, to which our utterances can even correspond. With roots as deep an ancient sophism and more recently associated with a school of literary criticism called postmodernism, this view implies that we should no longer concern ourselves with whether someone's statement is correct or not. We lack a standard by which to distinguish the true from the false. Instead the only determination we can make is whether the statement is sincere or not.

Frankfurt calls this an antirealist position, a view that seems to permeate many television talk shows. The antirealist says simply, "If we can no longer be true to the way the world is, because we no longer presume to know it, then at least we can be true to ourselves." The problem with this perspective, Frankfurt argues, is that it makes even sincerity itself bullshit. In forsaking truth and falsehood and aiming instead merely to be sincere, we are admitting that we no longer care what is true or false, which is the essence of bullshit.

What can educators do about bullshit? First, we must clarify in our own minds whether we think truth is a possibility. If all utterances are equally valid, then there is no point talking about truth or falsehood in the first place. Once we admit that there is some objective standard by which to assess the accuracy of what we say to one another, then we can take steps to rectify the conditions that promote bullshit. Next, we must cease expecting ourselves and others to render authoritative opinions on matters that we do not understand. We should make sure learners bump up against things they do not know. When they do not know something, they should learn to admit it.

This was the essence of the teachings of the prototypical philosopher, Socrates, who famously declared that he was the wisest man in all of Athens precisely because he recognized that he did not know. The quest for knowledge begins in the recognition of ignorance. If we think we know everything, or at least are prepared to act as if we do, then we are unlikely to learn very much. Instead of helping to clarify matters, we render ourselves polluters who merely cloud the understandings of others. We shed smoke, not light, and everyone suffers from our presence.

Ignorance is our friend, because it helps us to figure out what we need to learn. However, some of us are so insecure in our knowledge or so fearful of revealing a chink in our cognitive armor that, rather than admit we do not know something, we bullshit as listeners, too, by feigning understanding of any topic under discussion. We nod when we should question. This is a problem, both for the individuals involved and for the patients who depend on us. For one thing, it alienates us from ourselves, prompting us to live with a false image of who we really are. It also promotes a culture of obscurity in which it becomes harder and harder to distinguish between what we know, what we do not know, and what we merely pretend to know.

Far from fleeing what we do not know, we must, like Socrates, become connoisseurs of our own ignorance. Biomedical science marches forward not by converting the print already in textbooks to bold font, but by identifying what the textbooks got wrong, or even better, what the textbooks fail to address. To discover is to loosen our hold on what we think we know. If the renaissance Europeans had followed this path, the world might have gone unexplored. Instead we need to seek out and explore what we do not know. And those explorations need to embody a determination to distinguish with as much fidelity as we can muster the true from the false, the known from the unknown.

There is a vital difference between telling the truth and being truthful. In some situations, we may not know with sufficient confidence what is true and what is not. In those cases, we should be as truthful as we can. At times, we will be wrong. In other cases, we may be victims of deception. But we must be vigilant in our efforts to assess the truth of what we suppose we know. When we are wrong, we should be the first to admit it. In all cases, it is vital that we commit to veracity. From a professional point of view, it is more important to rescue the understanding than to save face.

Fostering Diversity

When we think about diversity in the admissions and hiring policies of medical schools, it is important that we carefully consider what we understand diversity to be and why we consider it a legitimate objective. Is it appropriate for medical schools to weigh candidates' race, sex, or ethnicity in such decisions? What factors should determine how different candidates are ranked, and should the underrepresented status of a group to which a candidate belongs play no role, some role, or a determining role in this process? What is the recent history of diversity in American medicine, and what arguments are presented for and against the use of race, sex, and ethnicity in admission and hiring decisions? Although grounded primarily in diversity as a factor in admissions, the following discussion pertains to diversity as a factor in selecting students and residents, faculty members, and staff.

Questions concerning the role of race in public education have been percolating in the US consciousness at least since the US Supreme Court's 1954 ruling in *Brown v. Board of Education*, which held that the 14th Amendment to the Constitution prohibits racial segregation in education. The issue of minority status in professional school admission decisions received explicit attention in the 1978 ruling in *Regents of the University of California v. Bakke*, when the Court stated that race could be considered a "plus" factor in admissio ns decisions aimed at achieving a diverse student body. The June 2003 rulings by the Court in *Grutter v. Bollinger* and *Gratz v. Bollinger* established that consideration of race and ethnicity in admissions serves a compelling state interest, but whole groups of applicants cannot be treated differently based solely on their race.

In a recent examination of affirmative action in medical school admissions, Association of American Medical Colleges (AAMC) President Jordan Cohen outlined the diversity gap in contemporary American medicine. Since 1970, the AAMC has recognized four groups as underrepresented minorities: African Americans, Mexican Americans, Native Americans, and mainland Puerto Ricans. Thanks to the efforts to promote diversity by the US medical schools during the 1960s, the percentage of matriculants from these groups increased from 2% in 1964 to 8% in 1971. Although the percentage of individuals from these groups remained constant for the next two decades, their absolute numbers continued to rise as additional medical schools were opened. However, court rulings in the mid- to late 1990s banning race-conscious admissions led many schools to curtail their affirmative action programs, leading to a general decline in the diversity of medical school classes since then.

Medical school admissions committees have traditionally relied heavily on such qualifications as Medical College Admissions Test (MCAT) scores and grade point averages (GPAs) in ranking applicants. Likewise, many residency program admissions committees rely on academic performance in medical school (GPA, honors, election to Alpha Omega Alpha Honor Medical Society) and National Board of Medical Examiners (NBME) examination scores to sort and select applicants. According to Cohen, medical school applicants from underrepresented minorities have significantly lower GPAs and MCAT scores than white applicants, and these indicators remain low even when adjustments for such factors as parental income are made. Explanations include poorer educational opportunities, lower expectations, deficits in parental income and educational experience, and a relative lack of support for academic achievement in some minority cultures.

Cohen estimates that if affirmative action were removed from medical school admissions decisions, the number of underrepresented minority students receiving offers of admission to the US medical schools would drop by approximately 70%, because of their lower GPAs and MCAT scores. With affirmative action, 11% of the US medical school matriculants in 2001 were from underrepresented minorities. Without affirmative action, the comparable number would have been 3%. On the other hand, the graduation rate for such students is 90%, as compared to a graduation rate of 96% for white students, indicating that despite weaker academic credentials, underrepresented minority students are generally able to "make the grade."

Let us now turn to the arguments for and against diversity-weighted admissions in medical schools and residency programs. Those opposed to racial and ethnic diversity in admissions decisions generally argue that the right of an individual applicant to be judged on his or her own merit outweighs any interest of a school or society in pursuing diversity. Citing the Supreme Court's ruling in the *Bakke* case, opponents of affirmative action argue that it is simply unfair to "say 'yes' to one person but to say 'no' to another person, solely because of the color of their skin." Every individual admitted to a medical school or residency program or hired to the faculty or administrative staff because of his or her racial or ethnic background is balanced by another individual denied admission because of his or her race or ethnicity. Does the collective interest of the state in pursuing diversity allow it to override the civil rights of a more academically qualified student, who will be denied admission due to factors over which he or she has no control? Opponents of diversity-weighted admission say no.

Opponents also point to the problem of defining diversity. Should African American, Hispanic, and Native American origin be the only categories of diversity, or should other categories enter into the equation, such as Arab origin, a particular religious affiliation, or being clearly Asian in appearance? What if it turned out that some so-called minority groups were in fact overrepresented in medicine, relative to their numbers in the general population? Should admissions committees begin granting preference to Fundamentalist Christian and Samoan applicants over

Jewish and Asian applicants, merely because the former are relatively underrepresented? If a history of discrimination is the relevant consideration, opponents argue, then Irish Americans, German Americans, Roman Catholic Americans, and Jewish Americans should probably receive preferential treatment, as well.

Another argument against diversity-weighted admissions is the fact that it generally makes all individuals in a particular group eligible for preferential treatment, whether or not they have in fact been the victims of discrimination in the past. For example, the fact that a particular student is black might confer an advantage even though he or she came from a background of wealth and educational privilege. Moreover, there is no guarantee that any particular individual would bring to the educational experience the diverse attitudes and perspectives that proponents of diversity-weighted admissions seek. For example, a particular black student may evince no interest in practicing in a medically underserved community, and may in fact hold political opinions that are diametrically opposed to the pursuit of diversity in admissions policies.

Opponents of diversity-weighted admissions argue that such policies fail to address the underlying problems that place many underrepresented minority candidates at a competitive disadvantage in the first place. Among such disadvantages are lower socioeconomic status and poorer elementary and secondary school education. Rather than perpetuating racial and ethnic prejudices in the admission process, opponents argue, concerned educators and public policy makers should be working to improve the quality of schools and the general living conditions in inner cities, where underrepresented minorities are concentrated. A number of medical schools have introduced programs that attempt to help individuals from disadvantaged backgrounds make up educational deficits through additional educational opportunities.

Another argument against diversity-weighted admissions is the fact that it has led many institutions to conceal their admissions policies. Wishing to promote diversity, yet aware that explicit quotas or preferences might run afoul of the law, some institutions have become reluctant to open their admissions policies to public scrutiny. Opponents argue that dissimulation and suspicion are no less harmful when they are being used to promote diversity than when they are being used to prevent it. They hold that admissions processes should be as open as possible, to avoid fomenting a sense of injustice that is deeply damaging to our society, and may even lead to discrimination against people who are perceived as having benefited from diversity-weighted admissions policies even when they did not.

Opponents question whether it is appropriate to redress discrimination through more discrimination, in effect disadvantaging white males today because of prejudice in years past against blacks, Hispanics, and females. They believe that such a policy would send the wrong message, saying that we believe it is appropriate to divide human beings into monolithic groups based on race or ethnic origin and to grant or deny them opportunities and resources on that basis. They hold that individual merit and equal treatment are more important objectives for a just society, and that granting particular groups special favors does them a disservice by suggesting that they cannot succeed on their own. They admit that race has been wrongly used in the past, but they deny that the solution is to perpetrate more discrimination.

Proponents of diversity-weighted admissions point to the growing diversity of the US population. For example, the US Census data indicate that between 1980 and 1995, the number of white Americans grew 12%, and the number of black Americans grew 24%, the number of Hispanics grew 83% (recently surpassing the number of blacks), and the number of Asians grew 161%. By the year 2050, it is expected that the percentage of Americans who are white will have decreased from 70% to just over 50%, and by the year 2100, it is projected that whites will be in the minority, at only 40%. Proponents of diversity-weighted admissions argue that the healthcare workforce needs to adapt to changes in the population at large, making it vital to increase the number of underrepresented minorities in medicine.

Do individuals from underrepresented minorities do a better job of meeting the healthcare needs of underserved populations? There is evidence that underrepresented minority physicians are more likely to choose to work in medically underserved communities than white physicians. There is also evidence that underrepresented minority physicians care for a higher percentage of patients without medical insurance or on Medicaid. Furthermore, there is evidence that patients being cared for by physicians from their own racial or ethnic group are more likely to be satisfied and have higher levels of compliance. Based on this evidence, proponents argue that it is in the best interests of the nation to promote an increased number of underrepresented minorities in medicine. It is also possible that increased diversity in medicine might promote more culturally sensitive research and healthcare management agendas.

Another argument for diversity-weighted admissions is the fact that some groups, such as blacks and women, suffered discrimination for many years. Consider, for example, the plight of blacks, as outlined by Cohen. Until the late 1960s, over 75% of black physicians in the US were graduates of only two medical schools, Howard and Meharry, and most medical schools graduated on average only one black physician every other year. In many cases, the problem was not that medical schools refused to admit blacks, but that the entire cultural and educational system conspired to prevent blacks from applying in the first place. Admissions committees were but the tip of a much larger iceberg of discrimination. Proponents of diversity-weighted admissions argue that this legacy of discrimination must be redressed, and that diversity-weighted admissions represent a logical and fair way of restoring balance.

Diversity-weighted admissions are seen by some as unfair, because they grant admission to less-qualified applicants while denying admission to more qualified applicants. In fact, however, GPAs and test scores are not the only basis for determining who is best qualified to practice medicine, or to enter a particular medical specialty. Proponents of diversity-weighted admissions argue that the purpose of the admissions committee is not merely to sort, reward, or select candidates based on their academic achievement. There is no law that says that grades and test scores are the only basis for ranking applicants. Proponents argue that other considerations are equally valid, and that among these other considerations are the larger healthcare needs of society. Medicine has a moral responsibility to serve society, and achieving a more diverse physician workforce constitutes a legitimate priority of medical admissions committees.

Building on this argument, proponents argue that societal interests in diversity are especially strong in fields such as medicine. Many proponents of diversity-weighted admission argue strongly for affirmative action in college and university admissions and throughout all the professions. However, because medicine is so intimately engaged in service to communities, and because health and disease are present in communities of every kind, it is especially vital that medical schools and residency programs produce physicians who are capable of meeting the needs of the diverse communities that make up our society. It may be undesirable that minorities are underrepresented among undergraduates majoring in such subjects as philosophy or linguistics, but it may literally put patients' lives at risk if they are underrepresented in healthcare professions such as medicine.

Finally, some proponents of diversity-weighted admissions question the validity of the traditional criteria by which candidates for admission to medical school and residency are selected in the first place. How strong is the evidence that GPAs and test scores accurately differentiate more and less qualified or deserving candidates? To be sure, the fact that they provide a quantitative scale for ranking is attractive, and appears to be more objective than simply relying on letters of reference and interviews. But does it work? Can we accurately predict who will become a leader in organized medicine, academic medicine, or biomedical science by GPAs and test scores? Can we predict who will become a great community doctor? The answer, of course, is that we cannot. Hence one might argue for a policy of using grades and test scores to establish a threshold for admission, but select among the remaining pool of candidates those whose overall record shows the most promise of meeting societal needs. In this latter determination, race and ethnicity, along with such factors as community service, ability to communicate, and general life experience might play important roles.

Medical educators, leaders in medical education, and medical students and residents need to give careful consideration to the issue of diversity-weighted admissions and hiring. By carefully considering the arguments pro and con, we can deepen our understanding of the questions at stake, clarify our own position on the controversy, and provide needed input as our medical schools formulate policies on this important issue. When it comes to the role of diversity in medical policies, there is no room for ignorance or apathy, because the future of medicine and the health needs of our communities hang in the balance.

Compensation

How much money should physicians earn, and what role should compensation play in influencing the professional decision making of medical school faculty members and our learners? This question is important to academic medicine for a number of reasons. Income is one basis on which college-age people choose their careers, and if physicians are underpaid compared to other occupations, medical schools may attract fewer applicants. Income also affects the choice of medical specialty, providing an inducement for students to enter fields that require relatively long courses of study, such as radiology and neurosurgery. This incentive is heightened when students emerge from training encumbered with substantial educational debt that they must begin to pay off once they complete training. Earning potential also influences where physicians choose to locate, as well as the choice between academic and community practice. Even within the ranks of academic medicine, income influences effort. For example, if clinical work generates more revenue than teaching, academic physicians seeking to sustain or augment their incomes may find themselves devoting less time to teaching and more to patient care.

Where you stand on physicians' incomes depends in part on where you sit. From the point of view of patients whose healthcare costs are rising rapidly, physicians' incomes may seem too high. From the standpoint of primary care physicians such as pediatricians and general internists, the incomes of specialists such as radiologists and neurosurgeons may seem excessive. Yet, to radiologists and neurosurgeons working longer hours in the face of declining reimbursements and rising malpractice insurance costs, incomes may seem barely adequate, or even insufficient.

A number of arguments have been advanced to justify the relatively high incomes of physicians. These include the fact that physicians contend with a strenuous selection process to gain admission to medical school and residency, undergo a long course of training, work long hours, face difficult decisions where life and death may hang in the balance, make major contributions to patients' quality of life, and so on. Of course, physicians are not the only people who work long hours, and some people barely earning minimum wage, such as taxicab drivers, work longer hours than many physicians.

Likewise, other groups in our society, such as law enforcement officers, face life and death decisions, but earn substantially less. The incomes of college professors are lower, despite the fact that many endure an equally long course of training and face stiffer odds of finding secure employment. Relatively poorly paid primary school teachers often make important contributions to their students' lives. If none of these conventional explanations explains the relatively high incomes of physicians, is there a rational basis for explaining how well doctors are paid?

Most analyses of physician incomes adopt a microeconomic perspective. Income is often regarded as a management tool, a way of getting people to do things they would otherwise avoid. If people are failing to do what we need, or not doing a sufficient amount of it, their compensation can be tied to their productivity in that area. For example, physicians could be paid according to the number of resource-based relative value units (RVUs) they generate. Such productivity-based compensation systems seem to offer some advantages. They mitigate the unfairness of paying low-productivity workers no less than high-productivity workers. They also discourage loafing and create a financial incentive for everyone to work harder.

Yet productivity-based compensation systems also entail perils. There is no guarantee that work effort and productivity are closely correlated. A physician performing procedures may generate substantially more RVUs per hour than a physician seeing patients in clinic, despite the fact that they are working equally hard. Moreover, such systems may underrate nonclinical but potentially important professional activities such as teaching, research, and service. Productivity-based compensation systems are also subject to abuse, if physicians begin to seek out high-RVU work and shun low-RVU work, potentially leaving some patients in the lurch. Finally, such systems can spawn a professional culture in which people begin to care more about the rewards of work than the work itself.

Compared to the microeconomic perspective, the macroeconomic perspective on physician incomes has received considerably less attention. From a macroeconomic perspective, the question is neither whether members of a particular group are being compensated fairly, nor whether a physician group's leadership is making effective use of compensation as a management tool. Instead, the question is whether particular medical specialists or physicians in general are being appropriately compensated relative to other workers.

Where should the incomes of family physicians stand in relation to other medical professionals, such as cardiologists, orthopedic surgeons, ophthalmologists, general internists, psychiatrists, and pediatricians? How much should physicians earn relative to people in other occupations, such as hospital administrators, nurses, medical technologists, public school teachers, college professors, firefighters, professional athletes, and the chief executive officers of large corporations? Would it be appropriate for medicine to be the highest paid occupation in our society? The lowest? If neither of these alternatives is appropriate, where should medicine lie on the income spectrum?

Psychologically, it is important for workers to believe that they are being fairly compensated. If people genuinely believe that the value of what they do significantly exceeds their compensation, then their level of commitment, both to their employer and to their profession, may wane. On the other hand, if workers feel that their compensation exceeds both their level of effort and the value of what they contribute, then their self-respect is liable to suffer.

Broadly speaking, there are four approaches to assessing the appropriateness of an occupation's level of compensation. These are market worth, comparable worth, societal worth, and fairness. Although none of these approaches provides a precise numerical formula for calculating the appropriate compensation for any particular occupation, each offers a distinctive and illuminating perspective. This section examines each of the four approaches to determining an occupation's worth, and then steps back and considers more broadly the standing of money as a source of professional motivation.

The first approach, market worth, may be succinctly summarized as follows: the appropriate level of compensation for any occupation or individual is precisely the income obtained in an open market for such services. According to social philosophers such as Adam Smith and Friedrich von Hayek, the array of factors involved in a thorough calculation of wages and prices is so complex and subject to so many biases that the free market is the only system robust enough to carry it out.

Suppose several physicians receive an offer of higher compensation to join another group. Should they? On the one hand, the new group offers a higher salary. Does that mean they automatically accept the offer? No. Perhaps the new group is located in a less attractive region, its reputation among patients is not as good, or the quality of its work environment is inferior. The market worth approach acknowledges that many trade-offs are involved in assessing the desirability of a position, and wages are not the only factor in the equation. When otherwise comparable positions differ substantially in their levels of compensation, prospective employees should ask themselves a question: why do some employers find it necessary to offer more?

There are limitations to the market worth approach. One is the fact that the US market in medical labor is not truly free, because the supply of physicians is constrained. The numbers of medical school and residency positions are relatively fixed. People who decide to enter the medical labor pool must devote many years to study and pass a number of examinations before being allowed to practice independently. There are also hurdles in the form of state medical licensure and board certification. If every person could decide to begin offering medical services at any time, competing with one another strictly on the basis of quality and price of service, the incomes of physicians might fall. From an economist's point of view, the professional requirements for entry into medicine artificially raise the price of medical services and the incomes of physicians. Some critics argue that such requirements represent monopolistic practices that redound to the detriment of the public.

Others believe such barriers to entry are necessary. They cite the profession's fiduciary responsibility to set high standards for its members and to police its own ranks. Can a layperson determine whether a surgical procedure is truly necessary, or critically evaluate the surgeon's technique? Can a layperson determine whether signs and symptoms are being accurately interpreted, or assess the validity of recommendations for management? Opponents of a free market in medical labor, including most physicians, answer these questions negatively. They assert that the general public lacks the knowledge and skill necessary to ensure quality medical care, requiring the members of the profession to regulate themselves.

Another pitfall of the market worth approach is the fact that it has the potential, over time, to turn professions such as medicine into mere businesses. To rely strictly on the free market to regulate practice is implicitly to adopt the view that the physician–patient encounter is fundamentally a commercial transaction. The physician is a vendor of health services, no different in principle from the automobile salesman, and the patient is a healthcare consumer, no different from a prospective buyer shopping for a car. On this account, the bulwark against medical malfeasance would be the principle that bad medicine is bad for business. When word gets out that a particular physician is taking advantage of patients for personal profit, or inflicting injuries on patients through incompetence, that physician's business will suffer. The market itself will weed out bad doctors.

Yet is this our vision of what it means to be a physician? Should physicians willingly prescribe any medication or perform any procedure for which a patient is willing and able to pay? Are physicians restrained from misconduct and incompetence only by their adverse financial consequences? Or do we believe that physicians should answer to a standard of conduct higher than the bottom line? Should physicians put the good of their patient before their own financial self-interest? If yes, then a purely free market approach to compensating physicians may threaten the profession's moral identity.

The comparable worth approach to assessing compensation rests on the premise that each occupation has an inherent value apart from its market valuation. The mere fact that people in a particular line of work tend to receive a certain level of compensation is no guarantee that their income is in fact appropriate. To take a rather extreme case, the fact that some individuals are able to generate large incomes through criminal activity does not establish that they deserve what they make. A comparable worth perspective might question some aspects of our society's current income distribution; for example, whether professional basketball players should be able to generate more income in a single game than a public school teacher earns in an entire year. Of course, another proponent of comparable worth operating by different criteria could argue the converse that the biological endowments and skills of such athletes are so rare, and their performances bring delight to so many people, that they warrant their substantially higher levels of compensation. It depends on the criteria by which we assess comparable worth.

What factors might enter into the calculation of an occupation's comparable worth? One factor would be the level of skill required by the occupation, and the amount of time and effort required to develop that skill. There is a positive correlation between years of training and the income levels of different medical specialties. No one would dispute that diagnosing disease requires a higher degree of skill than, say, sweeping floors. On the other hand, it is not given that performing medical procedures requires more skill than taking a patient's history, although the former tend to be more highly remunerated than the latter.

Another factor in determining comparable worth is education. The fact that physicians' incomes are higher than those of nurses might be justified in part by the fact that physicians undergo a longer course of training, and may be required to demonstrate a higher level of academic achievement.

Other factors that might be relevant in calculating an occupation's comparable worth include the level of responsibility assumed by its practitioners, the amount of mental effort required to perform it, and the pleasantness of the conditions in which the work is performed. On this account, we might expect the most highly compensated occupations to be those that involve a very high level of skill, a long and difficult course of training, great responsibility, considerable mental effort, and perhaps, relatively unpleasant working conditions.

The RVU system attempts to make judgments about comparable worth, although it is heavily biased in favor of activities that make extensive use of expensive technology. For example, a gastroenterologist generates considerably more

RVUs (and considerably more income) per unit time performing endoscopic procedures than counseling patients in clinic. Are we certain that endoscopy requires more skill? Is it truly more difficult or less pleasant to perform endoscopy than to take a complete history, or to educate a patient about therapeutic options? A truly robust system of assessing the comparable worth of different occupational activities would need to take such considerations into account.

Anyone advocating a comparable worth approach to determining compensation needs to address a difficult question: Who decides? Proponents of the market worth approach rely on the market itself to make such determinations, preventing any single person or group of people from gaining control over compensation. If we argue that the market cannot be trusted, then we must locate a person or group to which responsibility can be assigned. Should such determinations be made by a board of medical specialists, by the courts, by an impartial group of economists, or by representatives of the Department of Labor?

Some critics find it easy to argue that the salaries of certain medical specialists, professional athletes, and recording artists are out of line, or that different medical specialists, teachers, and law enforcement officers are underpaid. But to put such judgments into practice is a different matter. To accomplish that, authority for judgment and enforcement must be vested in some agency, involving a transfer of power with which many would-be proponents of the comparable worth approach find themselves distinctly uncomfortable.

The societal worth approach seeks to value occupations in terms of their contributions to whole populations. Such populations might be communities, cities, states, nations, or even all of mankind. From the perspective of societal worth, it does not matter how much a certain group of workers is being paid at the moment, or even how much they have tended to be paid in the past. Nor is it necessary to account for how much one occupation is being compensated relative to another. Instead, the critical question is this: how much does the public benefit from this particular line of work, and what level of compensation is appropriate to that benefit? Thus the societal approach adopts a fundamentally utilitarian perspective. It seeks to promote the greatest good for the greatest number of people, and treats compensation primarily as a tool for achieving that end.

A strong case could be made for the societal worth of any medical specialty. Consider, for example, diagnostic radiology. In a recent survey of physicians by investigators at Stanford University, cross-sectional imaging (computed tomography and magnetic resonance imaging) was rated the most important development in medicine over the past 30 years. Diagnostic imaging enables earlier and more accurate diagnosis of disease, more precise targeting of therapy, and spares many patients interventions, such as exploratory surgery, that they do not need. Diagnostic radiology is a vital component of contemporary healthcare.

Yet an advocate of the societal worth approach might ask some probing questions about a field such as diagnostic radiology. For example, how do we know that radiological services need to be provided by radiologists? Perhaps society would benefit even more were chest radiographs to be interpreted by specialists in other fields such as emergency medicine and pulmonology, and were neuroimaging studies to be interpreted by neurologists and neurosurgeons. Diagnostic radiology is important, yes, but is society making the best use of the resources it currently allocates to radiologists' incomes?

An illuminating way to analyze the social worth of a medical specialty such as diagnostic radiology might be this. What level of income would be necessary to entice a sufficient number of individuals to enter the field and promote a sufficient level of quality in their practice? Paying radiologists $1/day is clearly not enough. On the other hand, paying them a billion dollars a year would be overkill. In the latter scenario, many might opt for early retirement, thus depriving the public of experienced practitioners. Moreover, the associated reallocation of resources would have serious consequences for the rest of the economy. From a societal point of view, the goal would be to pay groups of physicians such as radiologists enough to guarantee readily accessible, high-quality imaging services, but nothing more, and certainly not so much that the community suffers.

Again, a crucial issue arises. Who decides? Services that provide little value to a population in aggregate may appear very desirable to small groups of patients. From a societal point of view, funds currently being expended on organ transplantation might be put to better use preventing diabetes, hypertension, and other underlying medical conditions that cause organs to fail. But to a patient in chronic kidney or heart failure, current levels of expenditure on organ transplantation may seem grossly insufficient.

The fourth perspective from which to assess compensation is fairness. The societal worth approach operates according to a utilitarian principle, seeking to ensure that compensation levels are set according to the greatest good for the greatest number of people. The fairness approach asks a seemingly similar but in fact quite different question: Are different occupations being justly compensated? Is it fair that a radiologist can generate more income in 5 min reading an abdominal CT scan than a primary care physician earns during a half hour counseling a patient in clinic?

These examples highlight an important feature of the fairness approach. Assessments of fairness always involve comparison. To make such comparisons, it is necessary to define a context in which they will occur. Such contexts may be local, national, international, or even cultural. Do we compare apples only with other apples, or with oranges and bananas, too? What seems fair in one context may seem distinctly unfair in another. The compensation of diagnostic radiologists may seem eminently justifiable compared to that of professional athletes. After all, radiologists are not merely entertaining people, they are helping to save lives. On the other hand, adopting a more global perspective, it may seem problematic to some observers that a US radiologist earns more money each year than many dozens of families in some of the world's poorest nations.

How widely do we set our field of view? Specialist physicians who are deeply offended by the fact that some members of their group earn slightly more than others may have no difficulty with the fact that members of their medical specialty earn twice as much as physicians in other specialties. Do physicians seek justice within their particular physician groups, or more broadly, in terms of the interests

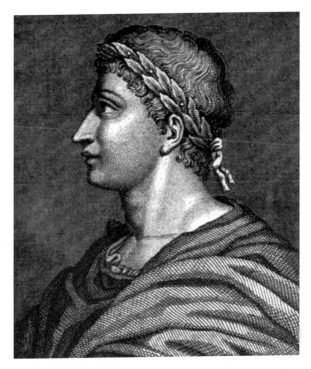

Fig. 7.2 Ovid (43 BC–18 AD). Roman poet who, in his *Metamorphoses*, tells the story of King Midas, a man who so loved wealth that he wished everything he touched would turn into gold. His wish granted, Midas discovers to his horror that his food and drink have become inedible. In a version told by Nathaniel Hawthorne, his inadvertent touch turns even his beloved daughter into a lifeless statue. Thus Midas comes to rue his wish. To what extent would wealth answer the prayers of future physicians? (Courtesy of Wikimedia Commons)

of their hospital, the profession, the society, or even all mankind? Twentieth-century moral leaders such as Mohandas Gandhi and Martin Luther King, Jr. insisted that we need to expand our field of view to encompass not only local interests, but those of humanity.

In Plato's *Republic*, Socrates contrasts two different kinds of physicians. One is motivated by the desire to make money. The other is motivated by a desire to improve patients' lives. The former kind of physician Socrates labels a "mere moneymaker." Only the latter does he recognize as a true physician. Where the good of patients and society is concerned, Socrates argued, true professionals must guard against the temptations of greed. According to ancient Greek legend, the Phrygian King Midas was granted his fondest wish, the ability to turn everything he touched into gold (Fig. 7.2). This enabled him to create as much wealth as he wished. Yet this apparent blessing turned out to be a grave curse, when he inadvertently turned even his own beloved daughter into a lifeless gold statue. Like the Socratic critique of mere moneymakers, the story of Midas serves as a powerful warning not to mistake suffering patients for goldmines.

No one would argue that physicians should ignore the financial aspects of medical practice. In fact, it is a good sign that many professional organizations are devoting greater attention to the business aspects of medicine, helping to place healthcare organizations on sounder financial footings. Such attention can remain salutary, however, only as long as physicians keep their gaze fixed on ends other than merely maximizing income. Are they using their knowledge of business to improve patient care? Are they helping to create a work environment where colleagues and coworkers feel proud of the work they do? Are they helping to advance knowledge within the field, and playing their part in training the next generation of health professionals?

What trade-offs are tomorrow's physicians prepared to make between earning money and helping patients? In the extreme, a purely income-driven physician might be tempted to increase patient throughput, and thus revenue, even to the point that quality care is compromised. How great a quality price are tomorrow's physicians prepared to pay in order to achieve a higher income? Alternatively, how much of a cut in pay would they be prepared to accept in order to practice better medicine? Of course, income and quality are not necessarily opposed to each another, but numerous situations arise in daily practice where it is impossible to maximize both. Taking time to talk with a distressed patient is often not the shrewdest financial move.

We need to ask ourselves and our students some basic questions. What would a practice designed to maximize physician income look like? Which functions would be performed by physicians, and which by other personnel? How much time would physicians spend talking to patients? How much research, teaching, and service, as opposed to clinical work, would go on in such a department? Alternatively, what would a practice dedicated to providing the best patient care look like? Which functions would be performed by physicians, and which by other personnel? How much time would physicians devote to talking with patients? How much research, teaching, and service, as opposed to clinical work, would go on in such a department? Of course, answers to these questions hinge in part on the time frame in which they are addressed. Are we trying to optimize performance for this day alone, or to build a sustainable strategy that would carry medicine forward for decades?

The compensation question is an important but by no means simple one. Few issues arouse more passion in the workplace, particularly when compensation is perceived as unfair. Yet there are many features of work life that are equal to or even greater in importance than compensation. Among the crucial questions to be addressed are these. Do people feel meaningfully challenged by their work? Do they feel that they are growing and developing, both as professionals and as human beings, through the work they do? Do they feel appreciated by the people with whom they work? Do they feel that their work gives them an opportunity to make a difference in the lives of others? Income is an important thing, but it is not the only thing. Where true professionals are concerned, it is not even the most important thing.

Where do we, as academic physicians, stand on the income issue? Do we believe that it is possible for a physician to be paid too much? If so, how much is too much? If we recognize no limit to how high physicians' incomes should rise, what are we saying about the role of money as a motive for medicine? Do we recognize other professional ends for which we would be prepared to trade income? What attitudes do we project to our students? Where does money rank relative to our efforts to deliver better care for patients, to advance medical knowledge, to educate the next generation of physicians, and to serve the profession? If we allow ourselves to become mere income maximizers, what will happen to the respect and trust in medicine of our students, our patients, and ourselves?

8

Organizational Excellence

We shall never know the truth for certain until, before asking how excellence is given, we set ourselves to inquire into the essential nature of excellence itself

Plato, *Meno*

Fostering Excellence

Medical schools and hospitals often spend huge sums of money purchasing and maintaining facilities and equipment, but relatively little time and effort attempting to understand the people who work with them. In fact, however, the single most expensive and certainly the most important item on the budget of many departments and physician practices is the compensation of the physicians themselves. The organizations alone do nothing. It is not the organizations but the people who work in them who make things happen. When something needs to get done, the crucial question to ask is not, "What lever should I pull?" but "Who can accomplish this?" In order to improve the quality of medical education we offer, we need to better understand the people who do the work.

We need to address some basic questions. Are excellent educators born or made? Why do some educators work harder and perform better than others? Can we predict which candidates for a faculty post will perform best? Are there steps that educational leaders can take to enhance the motivation of the people with whom we work? What motivators have the biggest effect? Which are more effective, "sticks" such as the threat of demotion and pay cuts, or "carrots" such as awards for teaching? Should we focus our efforts on placing our educational colleagues under tighter control, or should we attempt to increase their own sense of autonomy and empowerment?

If educational leaders do not understand the people we work with, the performance of our educational programs is likely to suffer. We will experience difficulties recruiting and retaining colleagues. Their performance will suffer, which not only threatens financial performance, but can adversely affect the quality of healthcare. The morale of everyone in the organization, including our own, may decline, because our needs and aspirations are not being taken into account in decision making. Failure to understand motivation compromises what the educational program can achieve.

R.B. Gunderman, *Achieving Excellence in Medical Education*,
DOI: 10.1007/978-0-85729-307-7_8, © Springer-Verlag London Limited 2011

One theory that beautifully contrasts different approaches to motivation is that of Douglas McGregor. He argues that there are two fundamentally different approaches to leadership, which flow from two very different views of human nature. One of these perspectives on human nature is generally negative, and the other positive. He calls these perspectives theory X and theory Y. Educational leaders who favor authoritarian approaches and prefer to work in organizations with a high degree of centralized control make the following theory X assumptions about people.

1. My colleagues dislike work and try to do as little of it as possible.
2. My colleagues will work only if they are provoked into it by direct control, coercion, and threats of punishment. Otherwise, they will show little commitment to the objectives of the educational program.
3. My colleagues have little ambition and would prefer to avoid as much responsibility as possible. Their principal concern is security.

As we would expect, educators and educational leaders operating from a theory X perspective tend to be highly directive, telling learners and colleagues exactly what they are supposed to do and extending to them little or no opportunity to participate in the decision-making process. When a learner asks, "Why do you want me to do that?" the response is likely to be simply, "Because I told you so." If a colleague objects, "I don't think that is very good idea," the supervisor might respond, "Well, I guess it is a good thing we don't pay you to think, isn't it?" Theory X leaders are not interested in building motivation or satisfaction, and helping learners achieve their aspirations is not a priority. Why? Because theory X leaders assume that we have no aspirations.

Theory X educators and educational leaders tend to regard others as tools (Fig. 8.1). We are seen as useful as long as we are doing what we are told to do, but eminently expendable as soon as we fail to bend to the will of our supervisor. For a theory X leader to succeed in such tasks as recruitment and retention of learners and educators, it is necessary to dangle very large carrots or brandish a very big stick. Otherwise, people will sense that the leader really does not care about us, and would just as soon be rid of us, if there were some other way of getting the work done.

Theory Y contrasts with theory X in a number of important respects. According to McGregor, theory Y leaders regard work as natural to us as play and rest. We are capable of finding in our work as learners or educators a great deal of personal fulfillment and often want to perform it for its own sake. External control and threats of punishment are not the only way to get us to do what is needed. When we are truly committed to what we are doing, we will display considerable self-direction. When the objectives of the educational program contribute to our own self-actualization, we tend to become very engaged in it.

McGregor rejects the view that we naturally shirk responsibility. Instead, he argues, we actively seek responsibility. When we seem inclined to shirk it, display little ambition, and seem concerned only with our own security, it is because our experience as educators and learners has taught us to, and not because we naturally see things that way. If we look carefully at our educational programs, we will

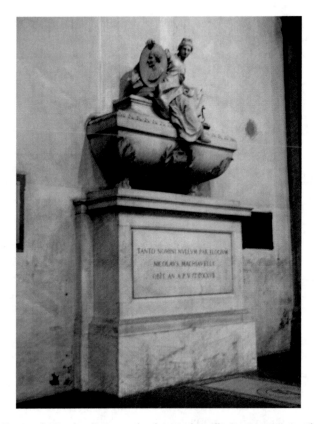

Fig. 8.1 The Tomb of Niccolo di Barnardo dei Machiavelli (1469–1527) in Florence, Italy. Machiavelli's most famous work is *The Prince*, a treatise on acquiring and maintaining political power, in which he wrote, "It may be said of men in general that they are ungrateful, voluble dissemblers, anxious to avoid danger, and covetous of gain." To say the least, Machiavelli seems to suggest, the prince should avoid thinking too highly of those he leads. Machiavelli's name is immortalized in the adjective Machiavellian, which refers to the use of cunning, manipulation, and deceit in the pursuit of power

discover that imagination and creativity are widely, not narrowly distributed, and much of the time, the intellectual abilities of the average educator and learner are only partially engaged. In short, most of us are capable of more than we are doing.

In contrast to the authoritarian theory X leader, the theory Y leader attempts to create work conditions that match the needs and aspirations of colleagues and learners. Where can each of us make a contribution for which we could be recognized? One of us might have strong information technology skills that could be put to work in developing and implementing new educational technologies. Another might be a good writer, and have a lot to offer in developing new educational materials. Still another might be a gifted classroom teacher, and perform best when working with learners in a face-to-face setting. A paramount objective is to involve colleagues and learners in decisions about how their work is targeted, organized, and evaluated, and to frame such decisions in terms of the larger strategy of the educational program.

Theory X represents a cynical view of human nature. It fosters an environment that health professionals, who place a premium on their own autonomy, are likely to find stifling. Theory Y, by contrast, holds that the most effective way to run an educational program is to respect and trust the people with whom we work.

Another helpful perspective on educational leadership is provided by David McClelland's "learned needs" theory. Applied to the educational context, it posits that each educator or learner operates with three fundamentally different sets of needs, which predominate to varying degrees in each of us. These needs are to some degree natural to us, but they are not merely inborn, and develop to varying degrees depending on our circumstances throughout life.

The first of these sets of needs is the need for achievement. Each of us wants to perform well in relation to recognized standards. We need to feel a sense of accomplishment, to help resolve problems, and to excel in our professional roles. The second is the need for power, the need of each of us to influence or control how others behave and to exercise authority over them. The third is the need for affiliation, our desire to be associated with others, to develop warm relationships with them, and to avoid conflict.

For many physicians, medical students, and residents, the need for achievement is strongest. Thus understanding and tending to this need is an important mission of any medical leader. People with a high need for achievement tend to prefer situations in which we can take personal responsibility for solving problems. If we find ourselves in situations with little or no influence over outcomes, we may become dissatisfied and lose motivation.

People with a high need for achievement also tend to set relatively high goals for ourselves. We are not trying to get away with doing as little as possible. We actually want to find projects that require us to exercise our abilities to the fullest. If our studies or work responsibilities do not provide us with such challenges, we are likely to grow bored, and perhaps to disengage. A lack of performance appraisal can be problematic for us, because we need systems in place that enable us to determine whether we are meeting our objectives. The need for power should not be equated with a need to control people merely to be in charge. Viewed in its most positive light, the need for power manifests itself as a sincere commitment to the success of the organization, and not merely a subterfuge of using the organization as a springboard for our own success. We want the course or the organization to succeed, and we believe that our influence with others can help promote this objective. We genuinely want to have a beneficial effect with the organization and the people in it. The need for power should be carefully attended to, particularly when developing and selecting leaders for an organization. If we ignore the need for power in those we educate and lead, it may foster the counterproductive attitude that they have no influence over others, which may leave them feeling useless and irrelevant. Such people will take their need for power elsewhere, in search of opportunities to play a more meaningful role.

The need for affiliation manifests as a desire to be identified with a group and to be well liked by its members. Those of us in whom the need for affiliation predominates tend to place a higher premium on the quality of our relationships than on our own accomplishments or authority. We may be willing to forego achievement and influence for the sake of friendship. This can cause problems in the realm of leadership where we want so badly to be on good terms with everyone that we find it difficult to make the tough decisions that our organization requires.

What kinds of leadership challenges are likely to prove especially difficult for the educator with a high need for affiliation? These include enforcing discipline, punishing infractions against the rules, and terminating employees. We may find leadership responsibilities very difficult to bear, because leadership calls us to types of interactions that we are temperamentally inclined to avoid. Similar problems can develop between the need for achievement and the need for power. Those of us with a high need for achievement may be among the most successful in an educational organization, but we do not necessarily provide the best leadership. We may, for example, tend to hoard responsibility, believing that we are the best qualified people to accomplish any task. This is problematic, however, because it means that the leadership abilities of others may be stunted, and because we tend to take on more than we can handle, working ourselves to death.

From an organizational point of view, it is vital that leadership responsibility be fairly widely distributed, so that we can draw upon the talents and experience of numerous people. High achievers tend to keep things to ourselves, but we need to do a better job of sharing if the educational program as a whole is going to thrive. In many situations, the individual with a high need for power may turn out to be the more effective leader, because we tend to think in terms of the entire group or organization, and to seek to lead others rather than do everything ourselves.

Victor Vroom has developed a theory of motivation grounded in what he terms expectancy. From the standpoint of expectancy theory, merely understanding what we need is not enough. We also need to understand the development of our expectations of how needs will be satisfied. He identifies three conditions that affect this decision-making process. First, we must believe that making an effort will change our desired level of performance. If we believe that it does not matter how hard we try, then we are unlikely to try harder. Second, we need to believe that improving our performance will help us achieve some goal that matters to us. Third, we need to value that goal.

From Vroom's point of view, we tend to view our daily work as more than an end in itself. We also see it as a means to other ends. He defines expectancy as our belief that effort will improve performance, and instrumentality as the belief that enhanced performance will enable us to achieve our goals. Hence, there are at least two levels of outcomes to which educational leaders must attend: levels of performance and levels of reward. The first level includes the quantity and quality of work we do, and the second includes the esteem of our colleagues, praise from learners and superiors, and promotions. We must believe that first-level outcomes contribute to second-level outcomes if we are to perform at our best.

Vroom also describes a factor he calls valence. Valence describes the value each of us ascribes to a particular outcome. One person might be relatively indifferent to salary, whereas to another, salary might be crucial. In the first case, salary has a low valence, and in the second, its valence is high. Thus, I could be certain that making a stronger effort would improve the quality of my work (expectancy 1.0), and certain that this improved quality would increase my compensation (instrumentality 1.0), yet care very little about earning a raise (valence 0.1). Because the three factors are multiplicative, a low value assigned to any one leads to a lower overall level of motivation, and I would be unlikely to make a greater effort at work because I had been offered a bonus. If we wish to motivate ourselves, our learners, and our colleagues, educational leaders need to attend to all three of these factors.

A key mission of leaders is to determine what second-order outcomes would most motivate us. If our compensation package is our greatest motivator, then we must devise means of enabling our colleagues to increase their incomes by increasing the quantity or quality of work they do. Conversely, if we are motivated most by a desire to make a substantial contribution to the education of the next generation of physicians, then we must seek out ways to help our colleagues make such contributions. Only by understanding ourselves and the people we work with can we optimally facilitate our pursuit of excellence.

As McClelland reminds us, however, we need to recall that our aspirations are not set in stone and may change over time according to changes in culture. We need to attend not only to what we expect today, but to the development of our expectations in the future. In an academic department, it might be prudent to avoid making compensation the premier second-level outcome, for fear that attention will focus increasingly on lucrative activities to the detriment of academic missions such as teaching that generate less revenue. We need to determine as a culture where the maximization of income fits into our overall goals for ourselves and our organization.

Because each of us does not share identical views on the rewards of work, we need to maintain openness to diversity and flexibility in our leadership style. It could be disastrous to assume that the motivational perspectives of a vocal minority apply across the board to the much larger and perhaps silent majority.

There is no single, universally accepted theory of how to foster the pursuit of excellence. Each of us and the organizations in which we work is a highly complex entity, and any effort to reduce our hopes and aspirations into a handful of factors is bound to introduce some distortions. Yet this is no excuse for neglecting the subject. Leaders in medical education need to be technologically savvy, but we also need to be wise people.

Do our colleagues and learners have the opportunity to do what they need to do? Does the organization provide them the resources to get it done? How well do our policies and procedures mesh with the abilities and resources to enable each of us to excel? By understanding what makes people tick, we can do a better job of making our educational programs hum.

What Makes Work Good?

Improving the quality of work has been the subject of scholarly research for decades. Thinking on this subject was stimulated by Howard Gardner, Mihaly Csikszentmihalyi, and William Damon, *Good Work: When Excellence and Ethics Meet*. The authors believe that "good work" can refer to at least two things. First, there is the quality of our experience at work and the contributions our work makes to our overall quality of life. Second, there is the quality of the product or service we offer. The two concepts are closely related, because if we take pride in our work we are more likely to enjoy it, and if we enjoy what we do we are more likely to do it well.

Gardner and colleagues criticize recent studies of work experience because they employ reductive or atomistic methods, confining themselves to breaking down complex work performances into elementary components. Examples in healthcare have included total quality management and continuous quality improvement. Viewing medical education from such perspectives, the final product might be students' scores on standardized tests, such as the United States Medical Licensing Examination. By analyzing the complex steps involved in producing a student's examination scores, we might develop strategies to reduce educational costs and improve student performance. These are laudable goals, and the quality movement has achieved important successes that have contributed to our educational programs.

Yet to really understand the quality of our work, we need to ask some additional questions. Why do medical educators do the work we do? What do we want from our work? What could be done to help us get the most from our work experience? Most of us feel better about our work as errors and inefficiency are reduced, but very few of us assess what we do strictly in terms of error rates and productivity. How do medical educators, and for that matter, learners in medicine, think about the quality of our educational experiences?

Gardner and colleagues encourage us to ask three fundamental questions. First, what is the impact of our work on the wider world? We need to see the work we do as contributing to life beyond our jobs and our organizations. If we do not believe that the world would suffer were we or our organization simply to disappear, then the probability that we will experience dissatisfaction and burnout is heightened. No matter how quickly or efficiently we do what we do, we need to feel that our work makes the world a better place.

Some might question this point of view, believing that Gardner and colleagues have set the bar too high. Is it not enough that we manage to perform our duties competently and provide for ourselves and our families, without enriching the wider world? In fact, however, people who excel at work frequently describe their work in such terms. They are not merely "punching a clock," when they set off for work in the morning. Instead, through the work they do, they are giving expression to the very best that is in them.

As medical educators, we need to ensure that our colleagues and learners enjoy opportunities to see the difference our work makes in the lives of others, and ultimately, in the lives of the patients we serve. Systematic efforts to assess educational quality can be helpful, because they encourage us to think about how our work can be more efficient or effective in an immediate sense, such as its impact on student test scores. Yet we need to keep a bigger picture in view, as well. Test scores are not the ultimate measure of our effectiveness, and we need to foster a culture where we can share our larger aspirations for work, where we frequently share with one another what a job well done has meant to us and others. An educational program that insulates us from the larger meaning of our work is asking for trouble.

A second vital question is this: How do we know when we are doing a good job? If the only indicators of work performance are throughput and test scores, then we are courting disaffection. Suppose, for example, that educators were evaluated strictly on their number of contact hours with students, or the scores of their students on standardized examinations. Does merely spending more hours with students necessarily translate into improved learning outcomes? Do standardized tests capture the larger vision of what it means to excel as a clinician, a researcher, and a teacher?

We need to expand our conception of good work to encompass not only narrow senses of quantity but also relevance, engagement, and our sense that we are performing at our best. Having someone with a stopwatch looking over our shoulder all day may in fact prove counterproductive, if it does not reflect the broader meaning of good work in the minds of those of us who are doing it. When we feel proud of the work we are doing, we find it more fulfilling. Thus we need to look for ways to help our colleagues and our learners perform at their best. Those of us doing the work frequently understand our work and the factors that contribute to its quality better than anyone else. Getting us actively involved in defining, assessing, and enhancing quality not only improves performance, but also proves rewarding in its own right, because we feel more of a sense of ownership in the work we do.

A third vital question is this: How do we become good at our work? If we adopt as our definition of work improvement minimizing the number of errors we commit each day, then we may begin to regard ourselves, our colleagues, and our learners as parts in a machine. This is a reliable way to discourage the best among us, because those who excel regard themselves not as interchangeable parts but as unique and committed professionals on whose distinctive contributions the whole organization depends. We should strive to create a culture in which we invest in ourselves, by encouraging ongoing education, enabling us to emulate the people we admire, and serving as role models to others.

If a group of medical educators feels that we are losing autonomy, the ability to control the structure and quality of our work, then our sense of commitment is likely to suffer. Likewise, if we feel we are being manipulated into increasing throughput at the expense of quality, some of us will begin seeking opportunities elsewhere. What seems like a good way to increase productivity in the short run, such as replacing live instruction with computer-based tutorials, may in the long run come back to haunt us, by compromising the many educational rewards that arise from contact with learners.

Where should medical educators who wish to improve the quality of our work focus our attention? Gardner and colleagues recommend focusing on what they call the three Ms: mission, models, and mirror. The mission of our educational program is the answer to this question. What are we trying to accomplish, and how does it serve others? If we do not know the answer to this question, we cannot perform at our best. When invited to discuss our mission, many of us feel both grateful and reinvigorated, because it helps us see more clearly what we are really doing. Deep down inside, we want to make a difference.

Even the most senior among us may lose sight of our mission from time to time. In general, this is most likely to occur in situations where we are overworked, in which substantial changes are taking place in the work environment, or in which we feel we have little or no authority in defining, assessing, and improving the quality of our work. In an educational program that is losing people, an attitude of survivalism may quickly prevail, and we may begin to see the program as a sinking ship from which we should take as much as we can before it goes under. We may start making decisions based on our own short-term financial or career interests, rather than the long-term mission of the organization. We may lose interest in longer-term efforts to improve the quality of work life, build future infrastructure, or enhance patient care.

To get our educational programs on track, we need to focus our attention on the program's mission and the role each person plays in achieving it. The best leaders are good at aligning the personal goals of workers and the larger mission of the organization. If there is a large discrepancy between the two, the worker, the program, or both are likely to suffer.

The second M is models. We need to interact with other people we deem worthy of emulation. Principles and techniques are important, but until we see them put into practice by real people, they remain too abstract for many of us. Role models are absolutely vital to every educational program, both for educators and for learners. We need to put a human face on the ideals we intend to pursue.

In an educational program that is declining, an effective leader needs to find admirable people and draw attention to their outlooks and habits. The goal is to get us focused on our shared vision of excellence, not to pick us or our program apart based on pet peeves and vested interests. Regular meetings are vital, because they allow us to discuss and reexamine our personal visions of what a great educational program should be doing.

Perhaps people from other programs that have surmounted the kinds of challenges we are facing could be invited to participate, sharing their experiences and recommendations. What were the key factors in improving their work? How did role models help people focus on the longer-term missions of the program? What pitfalls would they warn us against? It is good to discuss theories of work quality with educational consultants, but there is no substitute for face-to face conversation with peers who have confronted similar problems and opportunities.

The third M is mirror. It is vital that we pause from time to time to step back and examine the direction in which we are traveling. What kind of people and program are we becoming? When we look in the mirror, we need to ask ourselves,

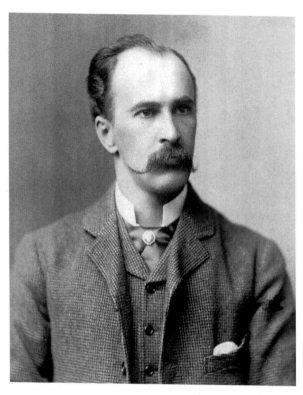

Fig. 8.2 Sir William Osler (1849–1919). Perhaps the most admired physician in American history, Osler served as one of the founding faculty members of the Johns Hopkins School of Medicine and later as Regius Professor of Medicine at Oxford University. Author of the most highly esteemed textbook of medicine of his day, he also introduced what we now know as the medical residency. Osler frequently emphasized the importance of character in medical education, and promoted the idea that "We are here to add what we can *to*, not to get what we can *from*, life"

"Are we proud of what we see? Would we be willing to hold ourselves up as a model of how this work ought to be done?" Many educational programs end up looking quite different from what we intended simply because we rarely take the time to look at ourselves in the mirror.

Winston Churchill is reputed to have said that we make a living by what we get, but we make a life by what we give. Making a living is important, even necessary, but we need access to far more than an investment portfolio to take the measure of a person (Fig. 8.2).

In reflecting on our work lives, we need to address these questions. What do the many hours we spend each week at work contribute to our larger sense of what we want to do with our lives? How do they enrich the lives of others? What can we do to make work more enriching for everyone involved? If we really care about the work we do, not because it provides a paycheck but because it enables us to make a big difference in the lives of others, we will enjoy strong intrinsic motivation to do it well.

Commitment

One of the most important factors in the performance of educational programs is the commitment of the people who work in them. If we are highly committed and for the right reasons, then our program is likely to flourish. On the other hand, if our level of commitment is low, a program is not likely to fare well, no matter how effectively its leaders function on other fronts.

Among the most important twentieth century investigations of commitment in the workplace is that of Frederick Herzberg. Originally, Herzberg studied approximately 200 rising accountants and engineers in an attempt to understand the sources of professional commitment. He began with two simple questions. (1) Think of a time when you felt especially good about your job. Why did you feel that way? (2) Think of a time when you felt especially bad about your job. Why did you feel that way?

From these interviews, Herzberg developed a theory that includes two basic dimensions of professional satisfaction, which he called "hygiene" and "motivation." Hygiene refers not to cleanliness in the literal sense, but to the healthfulness of the work environment. He found that both hygiene and motivation are important factors in a person's overall level of satisfaction, but the two differ in a number of crucial respects. Failure to understand these crucial differences, or to concentrate completely on either one to the exclusion of the other, invites trouble for any sort of organization, including our educational programs.

What Herzberg calls hygiene factors, henceforth here referred to as extrinsic factors, relate to the environment in which work is performed. They pertain not to the nature of the work itself, but to the conditions under which educators and learners are expected to perform. These factors include administrative policies, supervision, compensation, interpersonal relations, and working conditions. According to Herzberg, extrinsic factors do not enhance commitment, but failure to attend to them can severely compromise commitment. If we fail to keep our educational programs "clean" in these respects, even the best people in our programs may seek greener pastures.

One sure way to alienate educators and learners is to adopt policies that seem capricious or unfair. The sense of fair play is one of the most powerful sources of human commitment, and it is vital that we avoid offending it. If we feel we are being treated unfairly, our commitment to the organization's mission may disappear completely, and we may even find ourselves working against it. If faculty members feel that promotion and tenure policies are unfair, or learners feel that evaluation policies are unfair, serious discontent is likely to ensure. Nearly as harmful as unfair policies are unclear ones. We do not need policy and procedure manuals that are too heavy to lift, but people do need a clear sense of how the organization operates and how disagreements will be handled. We need to believe that our organizations treat us and our colleagues in a fair, respectful, and trustworthy fashion. We cannot afford to adopt condescending and patronizing attitudes toward educators or learners. An effective educational leader is not a prosecutor, but an advocate. The goal is to create the conditions in which our colleagues can thrive, by removing barriers to success and facilitating their creative efforts.

Another potential enemy of commitment is supervision. If we appoint as leaders people who are undeserving or incompetent, morale will suffer. We must resist the temptation to share authority only with people who agree with us, who can be relied upon to say "yes" to our plans. When that happens, we lose the opportunity to consider alternative points of view. We need people who feel comfortable disagreeing when they think disagreement is called for. Being surrounded by "yes" people only ensures that we become progressively more isolated and ill informed about our programs and the opportunities before us.

The same can be said for the assumption that the best workers always make the best leaders. In some cases, people who are very good at getting a job done may not perform well at supervising others who are doing that job. We may lack the desire or the ability to function well in a supervisory capacity. For example, we may find it very difficult to confront people with bad news, to delegate tasks, or to enhance commitment in others. If we aim to enhance the commitment of educators and learners, we need to be careful to ensure that we place in positions of authority people who have the necessary talents and perspectives to perform well in a leadership capacity.

We must also respect the ability of educators and learners to perform well without formal leadership. Medical students and residents do not always need someone to tell them what to do, and faculty members may perform quite well in the classroom without someone overseeing them. It is often the case that a group of colleagues can work together to address barriers and opportunities on their own, without someone looking over their shoulders. In some cases, appointing a supervisor may actually degrade commitment, because we feel that a vote of no confidence has been entered against us, as though we cannot bear the responsibility ourselves.

One of the most dangerous misapprehensions afoot in medical education today is the idea that we can enhance the commitment of physicians and educators through compensation. Herzberg regards compensation as a poor source of commitment. If we feel that we are unfairly underpaid, commitment will suffer, but there is little we can do to foster commitment through compensation. One way to avoid such problems would be to keep compensation secret, so that no one knows what anyone else is paid. The problem with such an approach, of course, is that we may share it with one another anyway. Moreover, secrecy by itself can over time undermine commitment, by contributing to an environment of distrust.

What is wrong with financial incentives for enhanced performance? One problem is the fact that we soon begin mistaking the reward itself for the enhanced performance the educational program is seeking to promote. We learn to care more about the reward we are receiving than the quality of the work we are doing. Moreover, we come to expect repeated escalations in the rewards being offered, and if that does not happen, we experience it as a punishment.

Another very important extrinsic factor in our commitment is the quality of the relationships we enjoy with our colleagues. One of the reasons we show up at work or school every day is our need for affiliation, to be with other people. In the best of all possible worlds, medical educators and learners feel a sense of mutual pride and camaraderie in our work and enjoy being members of our teams. We should be very wary of attempts to boost productivity by reducing break times and the like. Faculty members will not necessarily be more productive just because they have less free time, and students, residents, and fellows will not necessarily learn more just because they spend more time in formal instructional situations.

Highly educated groups of people such as physicians tend to become dissatisfied when we think that someone is trying to micromanage our time. This stems, in part, from the implicit lack of respect and in part from our resentment at being manipulated. Who knows better than we do how to allocate our time? Just show us what needs to be done, and then let us determine how best to accomplish it. There may be cases where someone needs to be disciplined for inappropriate behavior, but we need to do so in a way that promotes respect and even affection among our colleagues.

Herzberg also highlights what he calls workplace conditions. If we neglect the workplace, whether it be the faculty lounge or the classroom, our sense of pride and commitment to our work is likely to suffer. Facilities need to be kept clean and well maintained, and designed to be as warm and friendly as possible. Equipment should be up to date. Everyone in the organization should have some personal space, even if it is only a locker or a desk, and we should be encouraged to set it up as we see fit. In a medical school where space is often the most precious commodity, leaders may need to fight to secure adequate space.

In contrast to extrinsic factors such as policies and compensation, intrinsic factors concern the nature of the work itself. The key question is simply, "What do we do at work?" Attending to extrinsic factors can help reduce resentment and discontent, but it is primarily by focusing on intrinsic factors that we can actually make medical education more interesting and enjoyable.

If we are to be truly committed to our work, we need to believe that it is important and meaningful. If we do not care about what we do and see it merely as a means of killing time or collecting a paycheck, then we cannot perform at our best. As we have seen, one problem with performance-based systems of compensation is their tendency to shift our attention away from the work itself and toward extrinsic rewards such as salary and bonuses. As we focus more and more on the system for keeping score, we attend less and less to what we originally set out to do, educating the next generation of health professionals.

To help meet our need to feel that our work is important and meaningful, good leaders can help to ensure that we see its effects on learners, patients, the healthcare systems, and our community and society. Even anecdotes can be very helpful in this regard; for example, the story of how a young physician was inspired to pursue a particular medical discipline and went on to become a major innovator in the field. Collecting and sharing such anecdotes can deeply enrich an entire organization by reminding us of the kind of contribution we ultimately aspire to make.

Another intrinsic factor in our commitment is achievement. Some leaders are cynical, and believe that their colleagues are merely punching a time clock and care very little for the organization and the work it does. If this mentality becomes pervasive throughout an educational program, it can become a self-fulfilling prophecy of apathy and resentment. A far better approach is to assume that we really want to do our jobs well. From this perspective, our mission as educational leaders is to help educators and learners find genuine challenges that draw on their full talents and skills.

We need to keep growing and developing throughout our careers. We want to do well, and our educational programs can help us do so by challenging us to look at what we do and consider new approaches. Merely focusing on productivity in narrow terms can be problematic, because it may over time lead to a neglect of quality. If we believe that quality is being sacrificed merely for the sake of the bottom line, we are liable to become disenchanted and suffer even more serious declines in the quality of our work.

We see what we do, in part, through the eyes of others, and when we are doing our best, it is important to feel that others recognize our contributions. Such praise or recognition is another intrinsic factor in work commitment. Recognition means more than compensation, because it speaks more directly to our identities and roles as professionals. It touches directly on the work we do and what it means to us. It also highlights what our work means to our colleagues, our programs, and the people we serve.

We need to look for opportunities to recognize the people we work with for a job well done. This is not to say that we need to create employee-of-the-month programs, where an award is simply passed around an organization and thereby loses motivational value. A well-crafted note of praise or pat on the back is worth far more. Medical students, residents, and fellows need to see where respect and trust in medicine come from, and how important it can be to our sense of commitment to be recognized by colleagues and patients as experts with whom they enjoy a special rapport. This helps learners identify the kinds of relationships that will ultimately provide some of their greatest professional fulfillment.

Another factor in commitment is responsibility, a concept that can mean at least two different things. First, it can refer to ownership, our belief in and commitment to a task. Second, it can refer to empowerment, the authority entrusted to us over how we work. We are empowered by others, but ownership comes from within. It is nourished by participation in important decision-making processes and a belief that what we are doing really makes a difference. Herzberg emphasizes the need to give educators and learners ownership of what they do. If we practice what he calls "horizontal loading," we are unlikely to succeed at this. Examples of horizontal loading include increasing meaningless production targets, adding meaningless tasks to the work someone already does (such as preparing regular reports that no one reads), rotation of assignments between meaningless positions, and removal of responsibilities so we can concentrate on less challenging aspects of an already meaningless job. These and other forms of horizontal loading only decrease our commitment to our work.

Vertical loading, by contrast, involves removing external controls while retaining accountability. If we wish to deepen commitment, we need to avoid situations where accountability is high but personal control is low. Instead, we need to ensure that our colleagues enjoy as much responsibility and authority as possible for their natural units of work, such as a particular course. We need to make regular performance reports directly available to those doing the work, help them to devise new and more challenging assignments, and enable them to develop their expertise. The way to enhance motivation is to help the job—and ultimately, the mission it represents—become part of the person who does it.

Finally, we need to feel challenged by the work we do, challenged in ways that promote our growth as professionals and persons. The practice of medicine provides a marvelous opportunity to develop some of the most important human virtues, such as courage, honesty, compassion, self-control, intelligence, and wisdom. It is vital that we avoid eliminating such virtues from our educational programs. One way to invest meaningfully in the growth of medical educators and learners is to encourage and support self-directed education. We should spend less time telling our colleagues what they must know, and more time helping them to discover what they believe they most need to know.

Ethics and Excellence

Ethics is a complex and sometimes difficult subject, yet one of the most important areas of reflection and discussion in medical education today. It is not just a matter of rules. Of course, it is important that medical educators and learners avoid violating prohibitions against financial and sexual misconduct. Yet no one praises a person for merely avoiding infractions. Truly praiseworthy conduct, which also happens to be the most personally and professionally fulfilling way of living and practicing medicine, means more than obeying the rules. It means excelling at what we do, and helping others do the same.

The word ethics comes from the Greek root *ethos*, which pertains not to external rules but to internal character. The crucial ethical questions concern not what we do but who we are and who we seek to become. What is a physician? Are we highly knowledgeable and technically skilled body mechanics? Or is there more to becoming and being a good doctor than merely fixing broken parts? To understand what is lacking in the body mechanic model of medicine and gain a clearer and more comprehensive view of the ethics of excellence, we need to examine three levels of ethics. These are the impersonal, the personal, and the relational.

Though in key respects the least important of the three levels of ethics, the impersonal level is one that no medical educator can afford to neglect. It concerns such matters as organizational structure, efficiency, and finances. If organization is poor, even top people are likely to feel constrained and perhaps even doomed. In such circumstances, people see their efforts coming to naught. They are frustrated by the lack of resources to improve the physical plant, update equipment, and fairly compensate people. A railroad that fails to keep the trains well maintained and running on time will not attract many customers, and people will seek alternate forms of transportation.

Yet it does little good to keep the trains running on time if they are headed in the wrong direction. We sometimes forget this. We suppose that by getting the technical aspects of care in order, we have accomplished our mission. In fact, however, it is possible to attend so closely to one or more parts that we lose sight of the whole. We allow ourselves to become so entranced by enhancements to safety and efficiency that we begin to care for patients impersonally, neglecting the human dimensions of our relationships. We forget that, genuinely to care for human beings, we must first be human beings.

The personal level of ethics concerns what is taking place inside medical learners and educators. Behaviorism was a twentieth century school of psychology that encouraged us to treat human beings as black boxes. Based in part on the premise that we can never know what is going on in the mind and heart of another person, behaviorists argued that we should focus exclusively on how a person behaves. According to this approach, medical educators should concern ourselves solely with the behaviors we wish to extinguish or augment, and then apply the appropriate negative and positive reinforcements, such as salary cuts and raises, to produce the behaviors we wish to see. To increase throughput or decrease errors, for example, we should threaten pay cuts if standards are not met.

Such approaches are problematic because they are founded on a rather base view of humanity. Punishment and reward are not the only or even the most important influences on conduct. It turns out that what we do is really a reflection of a deeper and more enduring reality, namely, who we are. Many of us would avoid ethically suspect conduct even if we knew it could never be detected or punished. Why? Because our conduct reflects who we are, we want to act in ways consonant with our identity, and we want to be the best physicians and human beings we can. In fact, our conduct not only reflects but also helps to build our identity. We tend to become what we hope for.

To treat physicians as though all we care about is compensation, or promotion and tenure, or marching up the ranks of an organizational hierarchy is to treat us as less than we are. It presumes that all our motives are superficial, when in fact most of us long for deeper fulfillment in medicine. We hope not merely to get paid or promoted, but to be the kind of doctor we would want for our own parent, child, or friend. Avoiding infractions is important, but far more important is the call to excel at medicine, to practice it in a way that lives up to the aspirations that drew many of us into a career in medicine in the first place.

Good enough is not good enough. We want to be more than the kind of doctor that our patients and colleagues can live with. We want to be the kind of doctor that everyone can be proud of. This kind of pride—not vanity but genuine desert—is one of the most powerful motivators of human conduct. And it rests on a social foundation. We care about what we see when we look in the mirror, but we also care about how others see us. Will our successors be loathed and despised, or will they be respected, admired, and even loved? Is our approach to practicing and teaching medicine undermining or enhancing the relationships on which the profession itself rests?

At this point we move from the personal level to the relational level of ethics. Human life is an innately social, interpersonal, and relational enterprise. Yet it is astonishing how often we manage to distract ourselves from this fact. Narrow interests of productivity may lead us to organize our practices like prisons. We want physicians to be as productive as possible, which means seeing as many patients as possible, so we insulate ourselves to restrict the amount of time we spend interacting with those who count on us to care for them.

Physicians need to see ourselves less as wizards of knowledge or productivity and more as relationship builders. The notion that the candidates for medical careers are best assessed by their standardized test scores deserves careful reexamination. In selecting future physicians, we need to recognize the importance of building relationships and cultivating relationship-building habits and skills. To help prepare the next generation of physicians for these challenges and opportunities, we need to demonstrate the importance of such abilities, show that they are learnable, and reexamine medical education in their light.

A physician imprisoned in the impersonal level of ethics is a mere technician. A physician whose professional horizons also include the personal level can achieve true excellence and the fulfillment it provides, but only on an individual basis. To venture further into the relational dimension is to open up the full range of personal and professional excellence and to thrive by helping colleagues, patients, and organizations perform at and be their best. Where ethics in medicine is concerned, our calling is not to choose between the impersonal, personal, and relational levels, but to encompass all three.

Excellence and Failure

Everyone wants to succeed, but few people take the time to study excellence. Similarly, everyone dislikes failure, but few people invest the time and energy necessary to learn from their mistakes. Often we are too busy basking in the glory of our triumphs to think through what we did right, or the pain of failure is sufficiently intense that many of us want to "move on" and "put it behind us" as soon as we can. Yet those who want to improve their chances of excelling can ill afford to disregard the issue of why, despite seemingly equal levels of intelligence and education, some people tend to achieve at higher levels than others. The standard curriculum is absolutely necessary if medical students, residents, and fellows are to develop into competent physicians, but it is not sufficient to enable them to reach their full professional potential. A substantial amount of educational research indicates that how learners understand excellence and failure exerts an important influence on their level of achievement.

Medical educators would benefit from a better understanding of this influence. This discussion outlines ten parameters that tend to distinguish high achievers from low achievers, based on differing understandings of excellence and failure. These parameters are loosely based on a school of thought in psychology frequently referred to as attribution theory. Although some factors in the larger equation of achievement may be difficult to alter substantially, each of us can revise our understanding of what makes a person excel. In doing so, we can enhance prospects for excellence both for ourselves and the people with whom we work.

The factors that contribute to or detract from excellence can be divided into two categories, extrinsic and intrinsic. Extrinsic factors flow from the decisions of others, and include their expectations, reactions of praise or blame, and their choice of how to reward or punish performance. Intrinsic factors, by contrast, arise from learners themselves, and include their expectations, their level of desire to excel, and their sense of whether they were challenged in a meaningful way. For example, learners tend to feel a greater sense of pride in their achievement if the task they face is a moderately difficult one, as opposed to one they regard as very easy. Therefore, it is important to present learners with tasks that challenge them but do not overwhelm them. If they feel that they never had a chance, or that they did not need to push themselves at all in order to excel, they are not likely to benefit significantly from the experience.

Different learning environments can dramatically alter how learners perceive their performance and what they expect of themselves. If people are confronted with tasks for which they have no means of preparing, they are less likely to feel pride in their work, even when they happen to excel. Because learners are more likely to fail in situations for which they are not prepared, the experience of continually confronting tasks for which they lack preparation is likely to produce discouragement. Daily case conferences that fail to differentiate between first-year and fourth-year residents would be a classic example of this error. By orienting tasks to learners' level of preparedness, educators can improve their overall sense of efficacy as learners. Too often, the challenges and assessments learners encounter are not gauged to their level of training, and a sense of disengagement from the learning environment is the result.

By indicating to learners what is expected of them in terms of planning and level of effort, educators can further enhance their sense of learning efficacy. The goal should be to give learners a sense that they are in control of their own destiny. Fostering this sense need not be difficult, and yet many programs forego opportunities to do so. For example, medical students and residents should be given a set of learning objectives each time they begin a new rotation, and day-to-day questions and assessments should be tailored to these materials. This is not to say that learners should never encounter things for which they are not prepared. Such encounters should be a daily occurrence, but some balance between the two should be maintained, so that learners find their study reinforced with frequent opportunities to capitalize on what they are learning.

One of the traits shared in common by people who excel is a sense that they make things happen, as opposed to the feeling that things happen to them Learners who see the locus of control as lying outside themselves often see little correlation between their own choices and their level of achievement. When things go poorly, they blame it on bad luck, or on things other people did over which they have no control. By contrast, learners with a high sense of efficacy are likely to regard setbacks not as the immutable will of the fates, but as mistakes, from which they can learn and improve in the future. They study their experiences, failures as well as peak performances. Even when others contribute to their difficulties, they look for factors in situations over which they can exert some measure of control, and try to devise means to exploit them more effectively in the future.

Regarding the locus of control as internal does not, however, guarantee that a learner will react effectively to setbacks. Another key factor in how learners explain their successes and failures is whether they believe the internal factors are fixed or changeable. Learners who feel that their achievement accurately reflects who they are, and not external factors over which they exert no control, may nonetheless feel that their achievement is constrained by unalterable internal factors. For example, many learners regard ability as a natural endowment, something you either have or do not and can do nothing to change. Learners who interpret their failures as the result of their own intrinsic lack of ability are less likely to try to feel challenged by disappointments, and less likely to try to change their approach in the future. By contrast, effort is a changeable internal factor that the best learners attempt to improve.

People's explanations of how the world works and why things happen in their lives can provide great insight into their capabilities. The seminal approach asks people to recall personally meaningful peak performances or failures and to explain why things happened as they did. If a residency or faculty candidate responds to such a question with a look of befuddlement and cannot offer any coherent response, this is a good sign that they are not accustomed to reflecting on past experiences as learning opportunities. Similarly, if they portray themselves as innocent dupes or victims of forces beyond their control, this may indicate that they tend to experience events passively, rather than taking an active role in creating and influencing circumstances. By contrast, many people who excel tend to describe events as resulting from decisions they helped to make, and are likely to offer reflections on how they would do things differently in the future.

There is a difference between recognizing mistakes and labeling yourself a failure. In a sense, mistakes should be welcomed, because people who never make mistakes have ceased to innovate and learn. Rightly approached, mistakes are learning opportunities that constitute the stepping-stones to excellence. By contrast, labeling oneself a failure is likely to prove psychologically damaging and professionally debilitating. People who believe that they lack ability, that the tasks they face are too difficult, or that they have no control over the course of events in their lives are much more likely to consider themselves failures than people who interpret setbacks in terms of correctable deficits of understanding or effort. Perseverance, not genius, is the most characteristic trait of people who excel. In one of the most famous and briefest commencement addresses ever delivered, Winston Churchill encapsulated this lesson as follows, "Never give in. Never give in. Never. Never. Never. Never."

To say that people who excel tend to invite competition and unsuccessful people tend to shy away from it captures only part of the truth. There are two ways to win a competition. One is by choosing lesser opponents one can easily defeat. In choosing this path, people indicate that merely winning is more important to them than learning to perform at their best. By contrast, other people are primarily interested in doing the best they can, as well as helping others do their very best, and these people are likely to seek out challenges that force them to become better than they are. Comfort and fear of defeat can become enemies of human achievement, if they undermine the urge to take risks and push oneself to higher levels of performance. It can be tempting to attempt to insulate ourselves from competition in order to prevent the possibility of defeat, but people who give in to that temptation are consigning themselves to underachievement, and both they and their organizations are likely to suffer for it.

Three important characteristics of the learning environment that exert a huge effect on how learners set goals are the types of tasks they are assigned, the manner in which they are evaluated and rewarded, and the pattern by which responsibility is allocated. We need to assign learners tasks that challenge them at a level they can respond to and benefit from, neither too easy nor too difficult. We need to encourage learners to take risks, and to regard test scores and performance evaluations not as ends in themselves, but as means to the larger end of enhanced performance. If the only aspect of performance we ever acknowledge or reflect on is immediate triumph, then we may be encouraging people to sweep their mistakes under the carpet, and to forgo thinking about their work in a broader and more long-term perspective. Finally, we need to assign meaningful responsibility for learning to learners themselves, so that they become active and not merely passive inquirers. They should not require ongoing assignments from educators to continue to learn.

Some of the best contexts for learning defy our usual expectations as educators. We should encourage learners to work together in groups, with shared responsibility for learning. Such groups can be flexible rather than fixed, allowing members to come and go and to develop their own rules for learning. Because such groups can be small, they can tailor learning tasks to the knowledge level of individual members, creating a more efficient learning environment. They can turn the typically individualistic focus of medical education on its head, assigning learning tasks at the group level, thereby encouraging cooperation and mutual edification. They can provide truly substantive evaluations of what each member does and does not know and do so on a regular basis, rather than merely issuing a "report card" at the end of a few months or a year. Their goal is not to sort and rank learners, but to provide every member of the group an opportunity to learn. When they identify and correct mistakes, they do so in order to improve each member's understanding, not to determine who is the best. And they can ensure that each learner is an active participant who assumes responsibility for his or her own learning as well as that of every member of the group.

In order to achieve something, it is vitally important to understand clearly what one is trying to do. Learners who aim merely to avoid mistakes have sold themselves short. In such circumstances, learning becomes a byproduct of some other pursuit, and is likely to be less efficient and less effective. The best learners are the ones who seek out challenges and continue to question and grow throughout their careers. Just as learners need to understand what they are about in order to do their best, so educational programs need a clear vision of what they are trying to accomplish. By looking beyond the most immediate and easily measured parameters of performance and adopting a larger perspective that encompasses non-medical factors of excellence, medical education programs can prepare their learners to excel at even higher levels.

9

Center of Excellence

In shared activity, the teacher is a learner, and the learner is, without knowing it, a teacher—and upon the whole, the less consciousness there is, on either side, of either giving or receiving instruction, the better.

John Dewey, *Democracy and Education*

Sharing Knowledge

Professional excellence is difficult to achieve outside a good organization. Conversely, flourishing organizations are difficult to develop without good people. A domain where the intersection of professional and organizational goods is particularly important, especially in our information age, is the sharing of knowledge. If medical education is to thrive in years to come, it is vital that we become better knowledge sharers.

In medicine, sharing knowledge means more than developing new technology for transmitting and receiving information. A hospital information system may make information more readily available, but increased speed and wider distribution do not necessarily lead to improved care. This requires a kind of knowledge that mere information systems cannot provide. Likewise, a lecture may be enriched by the artful use of presentation software, but no technology can replace a gifted teacher who thoroughly understands both the subject and the audience.

Knowledge sharing is not just giving people information. It means collaboration in the pursuit of knowledge or its application. Whether the organization in question is an academic medical department, a family, a business, a university, or a whole society, its flourishing hinges to a substantial degree on the quality of knowledge sharing that takes place in it. This bears important implications for medical education programs and the people who work in them. We need to encourage our students, residents, and colleagues to ponder the meaning of knowledge sharing, why it is important, how it can be done, and what consequences are likely to flow from failing at it. Above all, we need to prepare tomorrow's physicians to share knowledge effectively. We, our organizations, and the entire profession of medicine will not flourish unless we do. This chapter explores the importance of sharing knowledge, with special emphasis on its pedagogical implications.

R.B. Gunderman, *Achieving Excellence in Medical Education*,
DOI: 10.1007/978-0-85729-307-7_9, © Springer-Verlag London Limited 2011

The world of human affairs contains two types of goods: those that can be protected behind walls and those that cannot. Among the goods that can be protected behind walls are food, land and other natural resources, living creatures such as livestock, and artifacts of various kinds, such as automobiles and gold jewelry. Some of these goods, such as food, land, and gold, are easily divisible: wheat can be sold by the bushel, land by the acre, and gold by the fraction of an ounce. In the marketplace, it is relatively easy to attach prices to such items. Other types of goods, by contrast, cannot be so easily divided up, and still others are essentially indivisible. For example, we cannot divide up and sell an animal such as a cow, at least not if we intend to preserve its life.

What kinds of goods can we not put in our pocket or protect behind walls? Such goods include knowledge, love, and power. It is impossible to capture the Pythagorean Theorem or the Golden Rule and secrete it away in a vault where no one else can get at it. Love lacks the physical properties of mass, color, size, and spatial location that would render it subject to hoarding. It might be possible to purchase a university degree, the outward appearances of affection, or even a particular political office, but procuring the outward trappings of such goods is a far cry from truly possessing them.

One of the most remarkable features of these intangible goods is the fact that, in contrast to food, land, and other fungible goods, they are not necessarily diminished through sharing. If you share with me half of your sandwich, you have only half a sandwich left for yourself. If you give me one of your oxen, you have one less beast of burden with which to plow your field. If you share some of your gold with me, your personal wealth is diminished by the exact amount you give.

The same does not apply to intangible goods. If you share with me what you know, your own knowledge is not thereby diminished. In fact, as educators well know, we often learn through the act of teaching. Sharing our love with others does not diminish our capacity to love. In fact, it enhances it, because caring is something we can improve at with experience. So, too, sharing responsibility actually increases the level of leadership in an organization, enabling leaders to get more done than would have been possible had they jealously hoarded all decision-making authority.

The distinction between tangible and intangible goods bears immense implications for the ethics of organizations and how we teach ethics in professional training programs such as medical schools and residency programs. Since we were tiny tots and our mothers insisted that we let other children play with our toys, we have been schooled in the importance of sharing. Throughout our lives, people who ignored the needs of others have generally been branded as selfish, and those who share with the needy have been greeted with praise and even held up as role models. Yet by the time we complete medical school and residency, many of us feel more concerned with protecting ourselves and promoting our own interests than sharing with others.

Maintaining a preference for generosity over selfishness in professional life can be difficult. Some practices of our educational programs militate against sharing. For example, the locus of learning in most courses and training programs is the individual learner. We gained admission to universities, earned grades, and progressed through successive phases of our professional lives largely as individuals. This tendency toward individualism is heightened by pedagogical practices that implicitly promote what game theorists refer to as a "zero-sum" mentality. If learners think that rewards are allocated according to a zero-sum system, in which the overall distribution of desirable and undesirable outcomes is fixed, they may begin to act as though they can raise their level of achievement only by outshining others.

An example would be a grading system that mandates a normal distribution, where every high grade must be balanced by a low grade. In such a system, each learner who does well makes doing well more difficult for every other student. From admissions policies to tryouts for teams to honors policies for graduation, such practices promote a spirit of competition in which every victory is accompanied by a defeat. The same might be said for organizational policies regarding hiring, promotion, and compensation, if they promote an attitude among workers that says, "If I am to win, someone else must lose."

These policies may implicitly encourage knowledge hoarding. In school, if a classmate of mine requests help with homework, should I be expected to provide it? After all, if I help someone else perform better, I am likely to shine a bit less brightly myself. If we are chosen and rewarded according to individual performance, why should we expend our time and effort helping others? On this account, we would do better to use our time to enhance our personal knowledge and skills. Each of us begins to see what we know as our own personal treasure, to be jealously guarded from others. Even if the sharing of knowledge does not diminish our personal storehouse of knowledge, it tarnishes its preciousness.

By changing our educational approaches, we can mitigate and even transform this implicit endorsement of knowledge hoarding. For example, we can adopt evaluation policies that encourage students to form learning alliances. Consider the example of learner-initiated study groups, in which learners divide up learning responsibilities among themselves, allowing different learners to study different components of an assignment, and then teach one another what they have learned.

In order to foster more cooperative approaches to learning, learners should be explicitly encouraged or even required to work together in teams, and evaluations should be assigned at the group level. Learners might also assume greater responsibility as educators. Groups of learners could be assigned topics to present to their colleagues, and the material they cover could be included in course examinations. Learners such as medical students and residents might even play a role in developing their own curriculum, determining what they want to learn, how they want to go about learning it, how they will demonstrate what they have learned, and how they wish to be evaluated. Such approaches help to promote a communal sense of responsibility for learning.

By concluding his *Nicomachean Ethics* with an invitation to read his *Politics*, Aristotle issued a resounding call not to attempt to do practical ethics in abstraction from the organizational contexts in which we are situated. Broadly speaking, there are two models of the organization, the authoritarian model and the participative model. An authoritarian organization is one in which decisions are imposed in a top–down fashion. The person or people in charge determine what the organization should attempt to accomplish, and then tell workers in subordinate positions what to do.

The problems with authoritarian organizational models are numerous. For one thing, lower-level workers dealing on a face-to-face basis with patients, families, and colleagues are not empowered to respond directly to problems and opportunities. Before presuming to do anything differently, they must first get permission from above. Moreover, the limitations of the people in charge become the limitations of the organization itself. Organizations can act only on what they know, and if the only working knowledge resides in a single leader, its knowledge base is necessarily narrow. Finally, the quality of knowledge sharing in authoritarian organizations is usually poor. We tell our bosses only what they think they want to hear, and soon all decisions are grounded in an unnecessarily incomplete view of the organization and its environment.

If organizations are to succeed in increasingly complex and rapidly evolving environments, we must enhance their effectiveness at collecting, processing, and disseminating knowledge. We need to become less authoritarian and more participative. We need to avoid establishing knowledge czars, whose very existence impairs everyone's access to reliable information. We need to enhance the incentives and infrastructure for knowledge sharing, thereby enriching the knowledge base of the entire organization. If people cannot see what the organization needs to know, have no effective way of disseminating what they are learning, or feel afraid to point it out, the organization will inevitably suffer.

We should see ourselves as members of a learning organization, whose products and services must evolve and improve over time. Firms manufacturing buggy whips in 1900 could not long survive no matter how much they improved the quality of their product, because the age of the automobile was dawning. Business colleges could not survive the twentieth century by perfecting a 1950s style curriculum based on typing and shorthand. What did people in such organizations talk about? What could have been done to improve the quality of their knowledge sharing?

Academic medical departments, corporations, and universities have become increasingly specialized. Accompanying that specialization is a tendency toward greater compartmentalization. The higher and thicker the walls that separate an organization's component divisions, the less effectively knowledge can be shared between them. An "us-versus-them" mentality often characterizes the relationship between the accounting and marketing departments of a corporation. Similar attitudes may beset medical school departments, hospitals, and universities, where we often allow the development of knowledge-hoarding fiefdoms. One of our greatest opportunities as organizations is to increase the permeability of our internal boundaries.

Consider the example of academic medicine. In most medical schools, faculty members can no longer adequately identify themselves as physicians, or even as members of a subspecialty such as internal medicine. Instead, we are cardiologists, endocrinologists, radiologists, and so on. In fact, even a designation such as radiologist is no longer specific enough: we are interventional radiologists, neuroradiologists, pediatric radiologists, and so on.

This has led patients to lament that today's medical specialists know more and more about less and less. Whatever gains we have achieved in depth of understanding have generally been paid for by losses in breadth. These costs of specialization are heavy. Consider what happens, for example, when a patient with complex medical problems is cared for by multiple specialists who do not communicate well with one another. Hospital stays may be prolonged, medications may interact with one another adversely, and patients may never get a clear picture of their overall plan of care. Failure to see the "big picture" can result in inefficiency, reduced effectiveness, and lost opportunities for synergism. We need to strike a balance between present comfort and future flourishing. High, thick walls that make us feel safe and secure today may render us irrelevant in the long run. In order to change a technique or learn an entirely new skill, we must be prepared to accept a temporary degradation in performance. In a world that continues to unfold in ways we cannot fully predict, where decisions must always be taken under uncertainty, we need to be prepared to take risks.

Merely exchanging information will not suffice. Deep knowledge sharing requires a willingness to subject our missions to the criticism of others, and to afford them the same courtesy. Consider the university. With each passing decade, the university more closely resembles a "multiversity," made up of distinct departments and disciplines that regard defending their own existence as their prime directive. In an environment dominated by turf wars, members of the faculty sometimes discover to our embarrassment that we have adopted an entirely defensive and reactionary posture.

In such an environment, we soon learn that questioning another discipline's reason for being invites unwelcome scrutiny of our own. Hence, we stop asking important questions. Inquiry into the fundamental definitions, missions, boundaries, forms of discourse, and standards of evidence that characterize different disciplines is stifled.

Such inbreeding and lack of cross-fertilization may promote a comforting sense of stability; however, they stunt the fertility of our organization's discourse. Creativity depends on diverse points of view, and such diversity is achievable only when a variety of viewpoints can be expressed. The most intellectually fruitful approach would be to create a culture in which sections, departments, and institutions are encouraged to pose serious questions to one another, and to expect serious answers.

This is a more robust version of knowledge sharing than merely presenting and publishing findings for colleagues in the discipline. Many of the most important contributions in the arts and sciences have been achieved by people working at the margins. Consider, for example, the crucial role played by physicists and chemists in elucidating the dominant biological puzzle of the twentieth century, the genetic code of life. In order to foster the diversity on which successful adaptation and innovation depend, academic departments, hospitals, and universities must learn to learn, and to share knowledge, more effectively. However, the intramural knowledge sharing that goes on within the boundaries of an organization is not inconsequential. This is particularly true if we realize that knowledge sharing includes discussion of the things we do not know. In terms of expanding and deepening our understanding, what we do not know usually turns out to be even more important than what we do know.

Our ability to make accurate predictions based on what we know is frequently so poor that we cannot even accurately gauge our uncertainty. Yet we would be mistaken to give in to the temptation to make an idol of certainty. When that happens, we simply keep repeating what we have already done. This presents us with a choice: we can continue generating results from the same familiar set of equations, or we can set about looking for a new and better set of equations. We need to redouble our efforts to cultivate a healthy skepticism in our students, residents, and ourselves. In cognitive domains such as medicine, the body of knowledge and intellectual worldview that serve learners reasonably well today will not suffice throughout their careers. Today's graduating residents will become obsolete within a decade if they do not continue to learn. Instead of merely memorizing the received wisdom of the past generation, learners need to become active inquirers in their own right.

No intellectual discipline is a mere collection of statements of fact. History is not simply the hypothetical card file or database that includes every single human event that ever happened. Internal medicine is not merely the sum total of all the facts in the internal medicine textbook, nor even the latest articles in the internal medicine journals. Instead, every discipline is an effort to interpret reality, or at least some particular facet of it.

Learners need to appreciate that even so-called sense data are in fact theory laden, embedded in a particular interpretive context. Our assessments of the hue, size, location, and state of motion of any particular object, or the very identification of a bundle of sense data as an object, reveals not only the percept but the cognitive context of the perceiver. Where a medical student looking at a chest radiograph sees many pulmonary nodules worrisome for metastatic disease, a more experienced physician may see unequivocal evidence of a benign remote granulomatous infection. If this interpretive principle applies to such elementary perceptual features as size, velocity, and benignity, how much more must it apply to the relevance of the ideas on which future innovation in the discipline depends?

It is vital that we situate our discussions of nontraditional topics such as ethics in their larger organizational contexts. Debating ethical principles in abstraction from particular life circumstances is not always valueless. Yet, it is only within particular sets of circumstances that practical ethical principles come fully to life. Those circumstances always entail institutional, social, and cultural contexts that define not only what we are doing but who we are.

It is all well and good to tell a group of physicians that we should protect our medical judgment from contamination by financial considerations. Yet we should not lead learners to suppose that the organizational context in which medicine is practiced exerts no influence. That context defines the very meaning of the phrase "financial considerations." For example, whose finances are we talking about? The physician's, the patient's, the department's, the hospital's, the health insurer's, the community's, or the society's? The level of granularity with which we explore the organizational context can prove morally decisive.

The range of alternatives apparent to the physician and patient is frequently defined in large part by choices that have been made in the background by neither the physician nor the patient. What pharmaceuticals are available in the hospital's formulary, and what are the usual and customary charges for a particular procedure? What is the moral responsibility of a radiologist who invests in an outpatient imaging clinic that "skims the cream" from the clinical revenue of a general hospital, forcing it to curtail some of its less profitable service lines, and thereby limiting services available to all patients in the community? If we are to prepare our learners well for the moral questions awaiting them in the real world, we must take careful account of such organizational contexts.

Finally, learners need opportunities not only to "talk the talk" and "walk the walk," but to examine the claims of their fields from other extradisciplinary perspectives. Consider scientific giants such as Darwin and Einstein, who famously enjoyed rather lackluster careers as students (Fig. 9.1). They serve as towering reminders that students who do the best job of memorizing the textbooks are not necessarily the same ones who eventually make the greatest contributions to a field. In fact, many of the most important contributions to a variety of disciplines, including medicine, have been made by outsiders. Who are our ship's botanists and patent clerks, our Darwins and Einsteins? Where are today's Harveys, Morgagnis, and Virchows, and what are we doing to foster conversation and collaboration with them? Far from diminishing, knowledge actually grows when shared, and the better we become at sharing it, the more cognitive synergy we are likely to achieve.

Encouraging Participation

The manner in which schools of medicine are organized deserves careful consideration. As the founders of the USA recognized, the ultimate fate of a nation hinges to a great extent on the structure of its government, and this is no less true of medical schools and universities. Medicine faces great challenges in meeting the growing demand for physicians, negotiating the murky and often treacherous waters of healthcare finance, and new ethical quandaries growing out of biomedical science, among many others. If we are to rise to these challenges, we need robust educational institutions and professional organizations that can help to formulate and put into practice appropriate strategies. A major factor in their effectiveness is the manner in which they are led.

How do our leaders attain formal positions of authority? Broadly speaking, they can be either appointed or elected. There are good reasons to think that a democratic and participatory process lies in the best interests of our learners, the profession, and the patients we serve. Given the magnitude of the challenges before us, it is

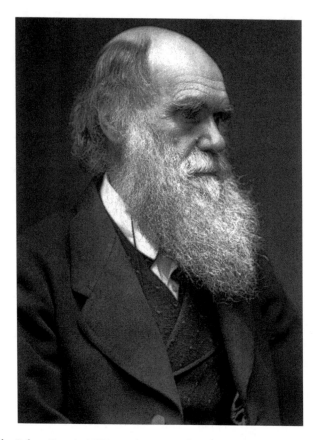

Fig. 9.1 Charles Robert Darwin (1809–1882). Born on the same day as Abraham Lincoln, Darwin failed to distinguish himself as a student at the University of Edinburgh, eventually withdrawing completely from his medical studies. Instead he pursued a career as a naturalist, voyaging around the world on the HMS Beagle and eventually formulating the theory of natural selection, which revolutionized our understanding of the evolution of life on earth. Musing on his voyage, Darwin wrote that "A republic cannot succeed until it contains a certain body of men imbued with principles of justice and honor." How can medical educators help to develop such principles in future generations of physicians?

now more important than ever that we avoid allowing leadership to become a merely honorific posting that requires little grasp of the larger issues before medical education. We are in trouble if leadership comes to be regarded as a mere rite of passage that naturally devolves on individuals after long and distinguished careers. At a time when adaptability and innovation are at a premium, we must avoid the temptation to control the process of selecting leaders and agendas from above.

One of the most important functions of any election is to give an organization's members an opportunity to choose. If there is no opportunity to play a role in the decision, or if the decision is presented merely as an opportunity for ratifying a choice from above, then the members have no choice. This can leave faculty members feeling disengaged from the medical school. Such a system of governance was more characteristic of the former Soviet Union than the USA. Medical schools and professional organizations should strive to ensure that our elections provide members an opportunity to exercise real influence. The choice of leadership should not be a mere formality, but should present a choice between two or more alternative accounts of our mission, vision, strategic plans, and goals.

There is no question that contested leadership choices can be awkward and generate lingering hard feelings among competing candidates and their supporters. However, few events would more engage faculty members and even students in the life of their medical school than an opportunity to choose between candidates who sketch out who they are and that for which they stand. The era when medical school deans and department chairs could be likened to museum curators has passed. If we pretend that we are still in it, our medical schools will themselves become museum specimens. We need leaders, faculty members, and students who are actively engaged with the challenges and opportunities before our organizations. Hearing candidates discuss the futures of our organizations and the profession draws us into dialogue and gets us thinking about our roles in defining and achieving their objectives.

It is vital that we eschew a "Wizard of Oz" approach to leadership of our educational institutions. In Oz, the person really controlling events stands hidden behind a curtain, pulling levers and turning dials in secret. Were faculty members to operate with the sense that the selection of leaders is the work of a group of wizards operating behind closed doors, then our interest in playing an active role in the lives of our medical schools might diminish. We might develop a client mentality, as opposed to a mentality of creativity and commitment. We might expect others to do for us what we could and should, for the sake of our institutions and programs, be intimately involved in helping to do ourselves.

Otherwise, we may find ourselves thinking like citizens of the former Soviet Union, who participated in the electoral process in large numbers because they felt that they had no choice, not because they were eager to exercise a right or opportunity to choose. That mentality distances members from leadership, and distances leaders from the membership. Were medical school deans or department chairs to feel that faculty members and students have little input into the processes of leader recruitment, selection, and retention, they might be less inclined to listen to what they have to say. If faculty members and students develop the sense that the only contribution they make is to pay tuition and dues, some might even be more likely to question the value of remaining associated with the organization.

A relatively close, top–down model of organizational governance is a prescription for a passive, uninvolved faculty and student body and a conformist paternalistic leadership. In the worst-case scenario, members may lose all interest in organizations over which they feel they have no influence. Leaders would, in turn, contribute to this downward spiral in participation by beginning to think and act as though the organization exists for them, instead of they for the organization. They might even begin making decisions based on what they thought was good for the leadership, as opposed to the good of the organization as a whole.

It is especially important that our educational institutions and organizations attempt to involve new members in leadership. It is vital that faculty members and students not spend their first years in a purely passive frame of mind, playing the role of people for whom decisions are made rather than people who play an active role in making decisions. By encouraging engagement in leadership and decision making, our organizations should serve as breeding grounds for future leaders, helping to develop the deans, department chairs, chief executive officers, and board members of tomorrow.

Elections can get us excited about what our organizations are doing. Every major decision, including long-range strategic planning, should be regarded as an opportunity to enlist members' knowledge, talents, and experience in charting the organization's future. We need to get leadership candidates actively committed to the process, encouraging them to interact with members and clearly formulate and express their vision of what lies ahead. Mistakes will always occur, but it is better to have candidates who attempt to craft a vision and fail than candidates who regard leadership as a caretaker role to which they have an entitlement because they are next in line.

Nonparticipatory models also tend to promote inbreeding, because each new leader tends to be selected by the preceding leaders. This can quickly render the organization's vision stale and reactionary. In the politics of leadership as in reproductive biology, mutation and recombination can have an immense salutary effect, by fostering creativity and producing a more robust organization that is better able to adapt and lead innovation in a rapidly changing environment.

Every leader choice should invite the input of the whole organization. If such choices become jealously guarded invitations to join a network of old boys, ossification will ensue. A far better metaphor for the leadership of our medical schools and professional organizations would be a laboratory of ideas, where bright people are encouraged to put forward new visions and strategies for the organization's future. Organizations that adopt such an approach can serve as leadership engines, fostering the development of new leaders committed less to protecting the organization from change than to putting the organization at the forefront of innovation.

This approach enables important challenges and opportunities to be recognized sooner, with more genuine discussion and debate over alternatives. It positions medical organizations years ahead of the curve of adaptation and innovation it would otherwise trace out. Junior faculty members need to view the leadership selection process not as a black box, but as a transparent and invigorating process that beckons them to become involved. The leadership of our organizations must not be separated from the people we most need to recruit and engage.

Getting More Out of Teams

The performance of teams is a topic of great importance to medical educators and future physicians. There are fewer and fewer solo practitioners in medicine. Most physicians work in teams, including both physicians and nonphysicians, where the performance of each member hinges to a large extent on the effectiveness of the others. Even physicians in solo practice often participate in professional teams of one kind or another, ranging from hospital capital and credentialing committees to local and national professional organizations. Most physicians also play a role one in one or more nonprofessional groups, such as civic and religious organizations. Finally, every physician has a family and a circle of friends. While much of the day-to-day work may be relatively solitary, as members of team practices, hospital medical staffs, and professional societies, we have a strong interest in understanding and enhancing team performance.

The ability of aggregates of individuals to outperform isolated individuals has been the subject of considerable attention in the business press. In *The Wisdom of Crowds*, for example, author James Surowiecki tells the story of a 1906 county fair where individuals were asked to estimate the weight of an ox. The total number of guesses was 787. While no single individual got it right, the mean of all the guesses was only 1 lb away from the correct weight of 1,198 lb. Of course, individuals operating in aggregate can also badly miss the mark, as recent dotcom and housing bubbles in the financial markets amply attest. Surowiecki argues that aggregates are more reliable when the individuals who make them up are both diverse and independent.

What interests us here, however, is not so much the wisdom of crowds but how to improve the performance of teams of people who are working together to make decisions. Consider another illustration that focuses more directly on the work of teams. A 2006 study by psychologists at the University of Illinois showed that teams of three, four, or five individuals perform better at letters-to-numbers coding problems than the best individuals. They attributed this superior performance to enhanced generation and adoption of solutions, rejection of erroneous responses, and information processing. Simply put, small teams tend to perform better than isolated individuals at examining problems from multiple points of view, generating multiple hypotheses, and critiquing possible solutions. Yet it does not always work out this way.

When people get together to solve a problem, there are three possible levels at which the team as a whole can perform relative to its best member. The team may perform less well than its best member. The team may equal the performance of its best member. Or the team may outperform its best member. What features and practices distinguish teams that perform more poorly than their best member from those that perform better? By understanding such factors, we should be able to achieve improvements in the quality of team decision making.

Of course, there are other benefits of team work beyond the quality of decisions, such as building relationships. In some cases, simply getting people together to talk to one another can produce important benefits in mutual understanding and respect, particularly when factors such as geographic dispersion and specialization prevent them from interacting otherwise. Team work can also promote cohesion, camaraderie, and shared pride in an organization. Consider, for example, a medical team made up of widely dispersed members who do not meet face to face except through their service on a departmental committee. In such a case, simply working together in a team can produce benefits as important as any particular decision the team might reach.

Other benefits aside, however, decision quality remains one of the most important potential benefits of team work. Even in organizational settings where a single person bears decision-making responsibility for the entire organization, it is still vital that the decision maker be able to draw on the insights of teams. Consider, for example, managing partners of medical groups whose partners expect them to make decisions on their behalf. Though many decisions may be made by a single person, the quality of the decision making still hinges on input from multiple people. If leaders do not listen to their colleagues, they will necessarily operate with less information than they could, and this can redound to the detriment of the whole team.

In an era of healthcare reform, it has never been more important for physicians to demonstrate the appropriateness of medical care in relation to utilization rates and costs. Many recognize the need for transparent, open-source, national appropriateness criteria. Though these should be grounded as much as possible in the best available empirical evidence, their formulation still requires team consensus. Diverse panels of physicians and nonphysicians who work effectively together represent key ingredients in the recipe for producing high-quality appropriateness criteria.

It is a mistake to think that the remedy for poor team performance lies in merely injecting more data into the discussion. Adding data to a defective team dynamic can merely amplify erroneous tendencies. For example, if the only data made available to a departmental committee come from a single forceful individual who views committee meetings as a mere formality for implementing his own decisions, then merely injecting more data may do more harm than good.

Empirical studies in the disciplines of political science, social psychology, and behavioral economics have demonstrated the difference a better understanding of team dynamics can make. For example, during the presidential administration of John Kennedy, lessons learned from the mishandling of the Bay of Pigs invasion were subsequently implemented during the Cuban Missile Crisis, enabling the USA to avert potential nuclear war. What steps are medical educators taking to help learners profit from past mistakes? Important experiential lessons could be shared within and across organizations, enabling others to avoid unnecessarily making the same mistakes while at the same time capitalizing on best practices.

The rationale for understanding team dynamics goes even deeper than this. Aristotle, perhaps the greatest mind in the history of western civilization, argued that human beings are naturally political creatures. By this he did not mean that every person belongs to one political team or another. Instead, he meant that every human being is born helpless and utterly dependent on others; that economic prosperity requires the cooperative division of labor; that we can only develop into full and mature human beings through social relationships; and that human happiness and flourishing hinge on the quality of relationships such as friendship and marriage. Teams matter to us not only in terms of our economic livelihood, professional authority, or personal satisfaction. They matter to us because, to a remarkable extent, our identities are defined by our membership in professions, communities, and families.

Often one or two members of a team know things that others do not. In a medical group, one member may be better versed than others in a subject such as economics, or have a better grasp of the needs of a particular group of patients, or simply know the parties to a dispute better than anyone else. Yet the person who knows more about one topic may know less about others. Knowledge and experience are distributed unevenly across most teams, and it is rare that the same individual is best qualified to address all issues.

When the members of a team pool their knowledge effectively, they know more collectively than any single person. If the members of the team are able to share such knowledge, incorporate it into decision making, and work together to implement it, then the team as a whole has the potential to outperform every one of its individual members. Of course, there is no guarantee that any team will do a good job of sharing knowledge, and the failure to do so is one of the most important pitfalls that teams encounter.

One way in which teams fail to share knowledge relates to confidence. In many teams, some members are more vocal than others. The people who tend to speak up early and often are not necessarily the individuals with the greatest knowledge and experience. In some cases, the most vocal members are not the best informed or the wisest, but merely the most confident. This can lead to problems, because there is a natural tendency for people who speak confidently to exert disproportionate influence on the other members of a team. People who know a lot but are not confident may contribute less than they should, or nothing at all.

Another factor that may silence people whose voices need to be heard is fear. Even knowledgeable people who have something to say may calculate the cost of gainsaying senior colleagues or contradicting the boss to be prohibitive. For example, junior faculty members or new members of a team who have not yet achieved partnership status may simply remain silent or even nod in agreement with leaders' points of view, despite harboring important reservations. This problem can be exacerbated in situations where the leader has previously punished people in some way for expressing dissenting views.

A variant of this muzzling effect is seen when members feel a strong need for affiliation and want to demonstrate loyalty to other members of the team. If everyone else who has voiced an opinion seems to be in agreement, or if the numbers on one side of an issue vastly exceed those on the other, people may feel obliged to express support for the majority point of view, even if they do not share it. Again, this tendency is likely to be particularly strong among newcomers who are trying to prove themselves good team players. Yet such tendencies are not confined to neophytes, and even senior members may always amplify the majority point of view.

These tendencies can prove disastrous. Suppose, for example, that a medical group's policies are formulated by an executive committee that consists primarily of very senior members who spend a relatively small proportion of their time doing clinical work. If an important clinical issue comes before the group, it is quite possible that most or all of the viewpoints expressed on the matter will be those of senior members who know relatively little about the day-to-day clinical affairs of the department. This tendency can be exacerbated when the few junior members still doing substantial amounts of clinical work feel reluctant to express alternative points of view, because they fear damaging their careers by contradicting more senior colleagues. In such circumstances, there is a danger that the policies adopted will poorly reflect the clinical reality they are intended to address.

The tendency of team members to go along with the views of others, sometimes referred to as a "cascade effect," can be quite pronounced. In most teams, there is a natural tendency toward convergence. Members tend to see discord as a sign of failure, producing a bias in favor of consensus. This bias can be so strong that it overcomes the goal of reaching the most appropriate decision. People want to be seen as good team players, or to reduce the level of tension in the room, or simply to conclude the meeting as soon as possible so that they can move on to other things, and so they go along. Instead of stoking the fires of debate, members keep things cool by keeping their mouths shut. Of course, convergence of opinion is not necessarily a bad thing. We naturally hope that many team meetings will result in a consensus. Yet, it is important to ensure that the process of reaching a well-informed consensus is not short-circuited by the cascade effect. The ultimate objective is not to reach agreement but to reach a good decision.

In some cases, a poorly considered and weakly held point of view may dominate a discussion, preventing alternatives from ever seeing the light of day. Or a timid member who tentatively speaks up may quickly revert to silence after someone else expresses opposition. This version of the cascade effect is likely to have been amplified, for example, when the final consensus opinion expressed by a team is stronger than the one that any individual participant would have felt was warranted. Everyone arrives at the meeting thinking that the team should opt for one alternative as slightly preferable to another, with plans to revisit the issue at the next meeting, but because of the cascade effect they end up proposing only one course of action as a "do or die" mandate.

What can we do to counteract these tendencies? One step is to ensure that teams are composed of diverse members. If every member of a committee sees the world in much the same way, then the potential of the team to perform better than any of its individual members is limited, because little mutually enlightening discussion can take place. Diversity does not just mean convening people of diverse ages, ethnic backgrounds, and skin colors. It also means recruiting people with diverse professional and life experiences. This is an important challenge to some radiology teams that are relatively homogenous in composition. If the goal of convening teams is to make better decisions, leaders must guard against the temptation to choose members who are likely to agree with them, and instead seek out people who really have something distinctive to contribute. In the long term, this means recruiting more diverse members. In the short term, it means making a greater effort to take full advantage of whatever diversity already exists. It may even require asking team members to imagine looking at problems and opportunities from the perspectives of teams of people who are not represented.

Of course, appointing diverse members accomplishes little if people do not speak up and share their distinct points of view. For this to happen, the rules and culture of the team need to welcome dissenting points of view. One way to ensure that every voice is heard is to invite each person around the table, especially anyone who has not spoken, to share an opinion. Another technique is to pause one or more times during the meeting and specifically ask if there are alternative points of view. And asking once may not be sufficient, particularly if some more aggressive members who have already voiced an opinion leap at the opportunity to say more. When one person tends to dominate the conversation, leaders can specifically ask the vocal individual to spend more time listening to what others have to say.

Another approach is to provide alternate forums in which people can express their points of view. Some people may feel reticent about speaking up in a team setting. When the decision at hand is momentous, the leader can make an effort to meet with such people one on one. An alternative is to encourage such people to express their views through email or internet-based chat rooms and blogs. Equally important is to provide opportunities for people to exchange perspectives in informal settings, such as around the water cooler or in the dining room. Such settings can foster a more relaxed and playful conversation that is more likely to spawn new insights.

Though it is always important to be sensitive to the feelings of others, it is important not to allow such concern to be carried too far. If the team is to make the best-informed decisions, people need to feel authorized to point out mistakes the team or its members have made. Of course, there are effective and ineffective ways of disagreeing, and it is rarely appropriate not to maintain a high standard of civility. It is almost always unnecessary to get personal. But people need to feel that disagreement is not only tolerated but to some degree expected.

The 1986 explosion of the space shuttle Challenger occurred in large part because NASA had developed a culture that placed accord above accuracy (Fig. 9.2). People who knew there was a problem fell victim to "Go fever," the attitude that delaying missions would only undermine morale and compromise the agency's political support, perhaps placing their own jobs in jeopardy. As a result, they kept quiet for fear that they would be seen as rocking the boat. In retrospect, their failure to speak up did far more damage than they could have imagined.

Improving team dynamics can enhance decision making. Consider in more depth the lessons the Kennedy administration learned from the Bay of Pigs fiasco and how they put them to use in handling the Cuban Missile Crisis. During the Bay of Pigs, the officials who attended White House meetings represented particular cabinet departments, and they tended to defer to standard protocols and recognized experts. Meetings included only a small team of participants who operated in extreme secrecy. Only a single plan was presented to the president, and no one was assigned to play the role of dissenter.

By contrast, during the Cuban Missile Crisis, more generalists were involved in the decision making, rank and adherence to protocols were deemphasized, there was direct communication between the president and knowledgeable lower-level officials, fresh voices were frequently introduced into the discussion, alternative

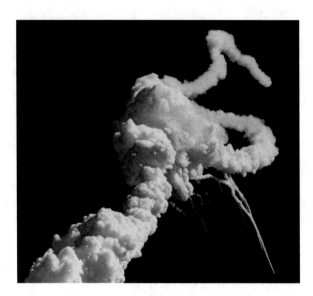

Fig. 9.2 The smoke plume of the Space Shuttle Challenger after its disintegration on January 28, 1986, which resulted in the deaths of all seven of its crew members. The commission that investigated the disaster determined that the culture and decision-making processes that had evolved at the National Aeronautic and Space Administration (NASA) were partly to blame. The agency had developed a bad case of "Go fever," at times allowing public relations to take precedence over the safety concerns of scientists and engineers

plans of action were presented, vigorous debate and critique were encouraged, and individuals were designated to play the role of "devil's advocate." The administration's superior handling of the Cuban Missile Crisis is largely attributable to the lessons it learned from the mishandling of the Bay of Pigs.

We want future physicians to be good team players. To support this goal through medical education, we need to change our concept of team players to include people who ensure that we see situations from multiple points of view and that each point of view receives a fair hearing. What each of us accepts without question or takes to be impossible may turn out to be otherwise, if we take the time to explore alternative points of view. We need to help medical learners to avoid seeing questions as personal attacks, but also to avoid challenging everything assertion simply for the sake of raising an objection. They need to learn to see those who challenge them in good faith as partners. And by challenging us, they are frequently doing us a great favor. Dissent does not equal disloyalty, and in some cases, the best dissenters prove to be the most loyal and valuable team members of all.

Educational Leadership

Education is the point at which we decide whether we love the world enough to assume responsibility for it and by the same token to save it from that ruin, which, except for renewal, except for the coming of the new and the young, would be inevitable.

Hannah Arendt, *Teaching as Leading*

Developing Leaders

The quality of medical education hinges on the quality of leadership in academic medical centers. Medical education programs that lack leadership, or are poorly led, are unlikely to thrive. In the effort to improve the quality of our leadership, we need to define the curriculum for leadership development. What do effective leaders know what skills do they possess, and what practical experiences do they bring to bear on organizational problems? What characteristics separate effective leaders from ineffective leaders? Merely having the will to lead is insufficient; we must also know how to do it, and bring the skills necessary to do it well. The essential organizational characteristics of leaders, the key necessities of their self-development, and the vital role of moral vision in effective leadership merit special attention.

Practically speaking, good leaders perform seven crucial functions in organizations. First, they affirm the organization's values. The values of a private practice medical group may differ substantially from those of an academic department. In the private practice group, most of the organization's resources are likely to be concentrated on providing high-quality, efficient, and cost-effective clinical service. In an academic department, on the other hand, other missions may rank equally as highly, such as securing research funding, publishing scholarly papers, and teaching medical students, residents, and fellows. Because such organizations cannot achieve visions they cannot clearly define, it is vital that leaders help to clarify members' values and do so in a way that people can rally around a common purpose.

A second vital function of leaders is to set goals. Members of many organizations operate with a sense of their mission, but they must also share short-term goals and objectives. For example, in an academic department, it may be crucial to secure extramural grant funding to sustain the research mission. In such a situation, a leader might facilitate pursuit of this goal by helping to develop extramural

R.B. Gunderman, *Achieving Excellence in Medical Education*,
DOI: 10.1007/978-0-85729-307-7_10, © Springer-Verlag London Limited 2011

funding targets that can be reintroduced at intervals to assess progress. This might include the submission of a certain number of completed grant proposals, and the use of such grant funds to help build vital infrastructure, such as personnel, equipment, and space.

A third vital role of the leader is to create and sustain trust. To work together effectively, the members of an organization must believe they can trust their leader and each other. The creation of such an environment requires open and regular communication. If organizational decisions seem to colleagues to emanate from a mysterious black box, then trust will suffer. Equally crucial is the style with which leaders react to error and criticism. A leader who reacts in a retaliatory fashion is likely to find him- or herself in a trust-poor environment where important information and perspectives are rarely shared.

A fourth vital contribution of effective leaders lies in the area of motivation. The members of organizations must believe in their missions. Unfortunately, too much attention is frequently focused on external rewards, such as salary and benefits. In a field like medicine that is rife with highly educated professionals, other aspects of work make an even greater contribution to our sense of anticipation and fulfillment in our work. A physician is unlikely to respond well to threats of pay cuts, and the value of annual bonuses is, at best, short lived and shallow. By contrast, a physician who believes that making fundamental changes in how an organization operates will enhance the opportunity to help patients, is much more likely to be open to change, and perhaps even to lead it.

Effective leaders also need to be good problem solvers. Even the best strategic planning cannot anticipate every contingency, and leaders need to be capable of responding to unexpected difficulties as they arise. The leader need not and probably should not bear sole responsibility for solving problems, for no single individual is likely to be able to see all relevant aspects of the problem or the alternatives available to respond to it. In a complex and changing environment, an autocrat is unlikely to provide effective leadership. Hence, it is helpful to involve other members of the organization, particularly those who are well informed and strongly committed. Ultimate responsibility rests with the leader, however, who needs to be effective in collecting information and perspectives, helping to outline alternative responses, and helping to formulate decisions in a timely fashion.

A sixth essential function of leaders is representing the organization. The leader is a flag bearer for the organization within the organization itself, the individual to whom its members look most to embody the organization's philosophy and ideals. Moreover, the leader represents the organization externally. If a leader is seen as inept, egocentric, or uncooperative, the whole organization may suffer. Leaders need to be able to articulate the challenges, opportunities, and vision of their organization in a way that contributes to the larger organizations of which they are a part.

Finally, leaders need to perform well as managers. Leadership involves the development and articulation of a mission and vision for the organization, as well as the motivation of its members to achieve it. By contrast, management means attending to daily operations, such as financial management and control, information systems, and personnel. In attending to management, leaders need to help maintain a focus on short-term issues, such as expenses and revenue. Operations are not as glamorous as strategic planning, but no strategic plan can work unless personnel and systems are available to implement it on a day-to-day basis.

It is a mistake to view leadership capability as something that is conferred on us at the instant we are appointed to a position of formal responsibility. Leadership capability requires the development of a set of knowledge, skills, and styles of interaction that encompass a personal philosophy. Peter Drucker has identified a number of important self-development tasks for all leaders and prospective leaders.

One of the key self-development tasks is identifying our own strengths. All excellent leaders tend to share certain characteristics, such as credibility, emotional stability, and good communication skills. But excellent leaders can also differ from one another in important respects. For example, some are good at sketching out a broad vision for the organization, and tend to leave its implementation to colleagues. Others are better suited to a more hands-on style, and thrive when they are actively involved in organizational management on a daily basis.

Some leaders do their best work outside their offices, thriving when they interact frequently with their colleagues, whereas others require a significant amount of isolated reflective time to perform at their best. Some leaders write particularly well, and others excel at speaking. Some love to roll up their sleeves for a good tussle, and others prefer to avoid open conflict. Some can thrive in a relatively unstructured environment, whereas others need a tightly regimented schedule to perform at their best. Excellent leaders get to know themselves well enough to know what approaches suit them best.

Once we identify the approaches that work best for us, we need to develop those strengths. Leaders who produce their best ideas through writing should structure regular writing opportunities into the work week. Leaders who perform best in face-to-face interaction should schedule the work week to permit a substantial amount of face time with key constituents. Many resources are available. One is the administrative team, which can be structured to complement the leader's strengths. For example, a leader who is good at formulating creative ideas but not so good at daily implementation would be well served by a staff that is more focused on operations. Leadership development programs can also provide important opportunities. These might include university-based degree programs in business, management, public health, and health administration, as well as nonuniversity-based programs focused more exclusively on different facets of leadership.

One key mission of all effective leaders is to overcome our own arrogance. We must avoid letting our fear of revealing our own ignorance create leadership blind spots. It is tempting to suppose that our long and intense professional training makes us omniscient, but a strong fund of clinical knowledge, research expertise, and excellence as an educator does not necessarily qualify us to excel as leaders. We need to recognize not only our strengths but our weaknesses, and learn to rely on others to help us promote the best interests of the organization.

Another essential feature of excellence in leadership is moral vision. Such vision is moral because it involves the organization's very reason for being, its highest aspirations, and it concerns vision because it involves what the organization hopes to look like in the future. To lead effectively, we must see where we are trying to go. Moral vision encompasses more than just a destination, however. It also includes the means the leader is prepared to adopt to get it there. Moral vision is reflected in the management structure of an organization, the style of personal interaction it fosters, and the incentive and reward systems it adopts. Ultimately, however, the moral vision of a leader is not a means to some other end, but an end in itself, the ultimate mission of the organization.

Moral vision may seem a less than vital feature of leadership excellence, until we consider the alternative, a leader who is either amoral or visionless. A leader who views the organization, whether a department or an entire medical school, as a mere tool for personal advancement is not really a leader at all, but a tyrant. Any attempt to operate an organization as a tyranny spells disaster for the organization and its members. Similarly, leaders who lack a clear sense of the organization's mission and their role in it have little business presuming to guide others.

Leaders who spend all their time and energy attempting to increase the efficiency of their organizations have lost sight of an even more important priority: effectiveness. Ultimately, striving to accomplish an objective with fewer resources is not as important as ensuring that we are doing the right thing in the first place. What difference does it make if the trains are running on time, if they are going in the wrong direction? What difference does it make if an academic medical department can reduce its fixed costs if the price is providing a low-quality education to fellows, residents, and medical students? Keeping the most important goals in mind is what moral vision is all about.

Ironically, one of the most important features of moral vision is the visibility of the leader. Members of the organization need to know who the leader is and that for which the leader stands. Ideally, the leader would have an open door policy, and colleagues would see the leader as accessible, open, and frank in communication. How can a leader who is rarely seen clarify the organization's course, inspire dedication, or generate enthusiasm? A phantom is unlikely to provide a strong moral vision, and thus likely to fail as a leader. We need to believe that we can trust our leaders and that our leaders trust us. To a substantial degree, leaders' authority rests on the sense of trust they inspire in others. By serving as an exemplar of trustworthy conduct, seeking quick, fair, and consistent resolution of conflicts, and creating opportunities to enhance our confidence in one another, an excellent leader creates a professional environment in which the whole organization can function more cohesively. Conversely, if members feel coerced into working harder by a fear of punishment, or bribed into it by the desire for some external reward, then trust and the dedication it inspires are likely to suffer. If leaders seem to waffle in their commitments or even renege on their promises, then trust inevitably suffers.

An excellent leader helps colleagues feel personally responsible for the organization, fostering a clear understanding of how their work fits into the larger picture. Ideally, each one of us should feel like a part owner, taking personal responsibility for how well the organization is regarded, both internally and externally. A sense of responsibility is nurtured when we give people greater control over their work, including active participation in decisions about hiring and firing, performance incentives, and investments in the development of human resources. Sharing information and decision-making responsibility, removing barriers and finding resources for others' projects, and recognizing and developing leadership potential all help reinforce our dedication to the organization.

A great leader feels guilty when colleagues do not have the opportunity to develop their abilities fully. We know when a leader is truly committed to our professional development. When we are treated as hired help, with superiors meticulously inspecting every aspect of our work, we are unlikely to be moved to invest our hearts in the organization. Autocratic leadership is especially ineffective when the people being led are highly educated professionals with a strong attachment to their own autonomy. By contrast, when leaders make substantial and visible investments in the development of their colleagues, they are much more likely to make significant contributions to the whole organization. The leader should not be regarded as an enemy, a policeman, a judge, or a jailer, but as a role model, a supporter, and a teacher.

When the interests of the organization require it, we must be prepared to relinquish some of our authority for the good of the organization. To someone with a strong need to achieve, there is something enticing about assuming responsibility for every facet of the organization's performance. It gives us greater control, and accords us more of the credit when our efforts succeed. However, no single person can take responsibility for every aspect of a complex organization. The delegation and diffusion of responsibility and authority are vital if colleagues are to realize their full potential. Leaders need not exercise iron-fisted control over every decision in order to be respected or valued as leaders.

Understanding Leadership

Perhaps the most important characteristic of an effective leader is a clear sense of where the group or organization should be headed. It is difficult, if not impossible, truly to lead other people when we ourselves have no route or destination in mind. That being said, however, there is much more to effective leadership in medical education than a vision of what the program should look like in the future and a strong sense of mission: why it exists in the first place. For the last few decades, many investigators in the field have approached leadership less as a specific set of goals and more in terms of the influence of the leader. A good deal of research in the social sciences has focused on two factors in the leadership equation: the leader and the organization.

The personality and conduct of leaders are crucial factors in understanding how effective leadership is possible. Leaders and followers generally think differently from one another, and there are important differences between those who succeed as leaders and those who fail. By exploring these differences, we can illuminate the characteristics of effective leadership and develop better leaders. Yet leadership never works in a vacuum. The effectiveness of leaders is powerfully affected by the nature of the organization in which we operate. What works well in one situation may fail miserably in another.

In attempting to catalogue the personal characteristics of leaders, investigators have grouped key personality traits into three categories: intelligence, personality, and interpersonal abilities. In terms of intelligence, leaders tend to display greater ability than followers in terms of the breadth and depth of their knowledge base concerning people and organizations, their decisiveness, and their fluency of communication. In terms of personality, they tend to be alert, creative, self-confident, self-controlled, and independent, sometimes even to the point of nonconformity. Their interpersonal abilities include sociability, tact, a greater-than-normal capacity for enlisting cooperation, and a generally elevated level of popularity and prestige.

What personality traits make up a good leader in medical education, and how can we determine who among us has the most potential to excel as a leader? In many respects, a generic answer grounded in intelligence, personality, and interpersonal abilities will suffice. For example, an individual who does not enjoy working with other people or who has little interest in how organizations function would be a poor choice to lead a department or a medical school, no matter how effective that person might be as a classroom teacher, clinician, or researcher. The person best suited to lead will not always be the best in any of these other respects, although it is important to understand what excellence in those activities entails and to be committed to helping others achieve it. Research into the personal aspects of leadership provides insights into the leadership prospects of different individuals. Yet such a profile says little about what leaders in fact do. In what ways does the behavior of leaders differ from that of followers, and can we arrive at any generalizations about the patterns of conduct of leaders that are most effective?

Large studies conducted at Ohio State University and Michigan University after the Second World War shed important light on this aspect of leadership. Personality may be difficult, perhaps even impossible to change, but most of us can change our patterns of conduct to some degree, and thereby lead more effectively.

The Ohio State studies emphasize two key aspects of leadership conduct: consideration and initiating structure. Consideration is the degree to which leaders show concern for subordinates, act in a congenial manner, and look out for the welfare of members of the organization. Initiating structure is the degree to which the leader helps to define roles that are structured toward the attainment of the organization's goals. Initial attempts to define such patterns of conduct place consideration and initiating structure at opposite ends of a spectrum, but subsequent research has indicated that the most effective leaders score highly in both areas.

The University of Michigan group distinguished between styles of leadership that are job centered and those that are employee centered. Job-centered leaders tend to emphasize the technical or formal aspects of jobs and to view colleagues as means of achieving the organization's ends. By contrast, employee-centered leaders tend to emphasize interpersonal relations, making the personal needs of colleagues a priority, and welcoming personality differences between members of the organization. Again, subsequent investigation has tended to indicate that the best leaders manifest both job-centered and employee-centered approaches to leadership.

Renesis Likert at Michigan elaborated these early studies into a more complex model of the conduct of leaders, based on four styles of interpersonal relations that he called the autocratic, the benevolent, the consultative, and the participatory.

The autocratic style is characterized by unilateral decision making, legitimated by the formal authority granted by the organization. Autocratic department chairs or deans would tend to make decisions without seeking the advice or consent of colleagues, relying on their formal authority to validate and implement changes. The autocratic leader is not particularly concerned for the psychological or professional welfare of subordinates, and those who oppose the autocrat's will are likely to be disciplined or even discharged. Conversely, those who cooperate with the autocrat's edicts may be rewarded, but only in formal organizational terms, such as salary raises and promotions.

The benevolent style is characterized by an interest and trust in colleagues, but decision making itself remains authoritarian. In contrast to the autocrat, the benevolent leader wants followers to be happy and successful, but like the autocrat, does not involve others in the decision making. If the autocrat can be conceptualized as the worst type of military leader who regards those in the chain of command as interchangeable parts in a machine, the benevolent leader can be conceptualized in parental terms. In these respects, both autocratic and benevolent leaders may be viewed by others as excessively restrictive or even demeaning, particularly if we believe we are capable of making an important contribution to decision making.

Consultative leaders involve others in decision making, although they do not rely on consensus building to implement change. A consultative leader invites both formal and informal advice from others, attempting to glean as much insight as possible from knowledgeable and concerned parties as possible. However, the decision itself always rests with the leader, with the expectation that others will comply whether they are ultimately in agreement or not.

The participatory style of leadership entails the highest level of subordinate involvement in decision making, with reciprocal and even mutual relationships between leaders and their colleagues. It represents a fundamentally democratic approach in which we are prized not only for the quality of knowledge we can contribute to decision making, but for our ability to help achieve consensus. Members of the organization must exhibit a substantial degree of maturity and willingness to bear responsibility for making and implementing decisions if this leadership style is to be effective.

The performance of the participatory style often exceeds that of the others. In participatory settings, followers tend to identify more closely with the organization, having helped to set its priorities. Moreover, participation enhances the personal growth and development of a program's members, which contributes to the leadership development of others. Participation also fosters the growth of a marketplace of ideas, bringing to bear a more varied range of perspectives and insights than that expected with less participatory styles of leadership. Finally, decisions reached through a participatory process tend to meet with less resistance, thereby facilitating change. In general, groups of highly educated individuals such as medical educators are likely to respond best to more participatory styles, at least where the issues at stake are ones in which they would want to play a role in decision making.

Another area of research into leadership concerns power itself. This has less to do with the relationship between leaders and colleagues and more to do with that between leaders and organizations, from which power to some degree derives. In crude terms, leaders are generally the people in an organization who wield the most power, manifesting the greatest capacity to influence the ideas and actions of others. French and Raven described five bases of power: legitimate power, reward power, coercive power, expert power, and referent power. Legitimate power derives from our position in the organization. Department chairs enjoy a certain amount of influence over the decisions and actions of others simply because they are the chair. Of course, the strength of a chair's power will vary from institution to institution, depending on the particular management structure in place. For example, chairs are likely to enjoy greater legitimate power in institutions where personnel decisions such as hiring and firing are largely within the chair's control.

Reward power arises from the leader's ability to compensate others for desirable conduct. Chairs are likely to enjoy more power in departments where they enjoy great discretion in distributing such rewards as salary raises, promotions, and desirable work schedules. In fields such as medicine and medical education, even purely honorific rewards may be highly coveted.

Coercive power refers to leaders' ability to punish others for undesirable conduct, either through direct sanctions or the withholding of rewards (Fig. 10.1). Chairs and deans are more powerful when they are able unilaterally to punish colleagues by reducing salaries, withholding salary increases, denying or delaying promotion and tenure, assigning unpleasant or unrewarding tasks, and so on. Great political theorists such as Thucydides and Machiavelli repeatedly emphasize the importance of coercion not only as an instrument of power already acquired, but a means of garnering and consolidating power. Among physicians and medical educators, however, regular recourse to coercion is likely to undercut organizational morale and may ultimately diminish the authority of the leader.

Expert power derives from the leader's ability to influence others because of special knowledge or skills important to the organization's mission. This power is the personal possession of the person who wields it and cannot be directly bestowed by the organization or its management structure. In this respect, it differs from legitimate power, reward power, and coercive power. Types of expert power among medical educators include the knowledge and skills that make a good medical educator. Even more important to leaders, however, are the leadership knowledge and skills that make a medical educator not merely a good physician or scientist, but a good leader.

Like expert power, referent power cannot be bestowed by the organization. It involves the admiration and loyalty that we earn through our interactions with others, and in particular, through our ability to lead by example. The German sociologist Max Weber used the term "charisma" to describe this kind of leader. Charismatic chairs or deans are not only naturally magnetic individuals, but

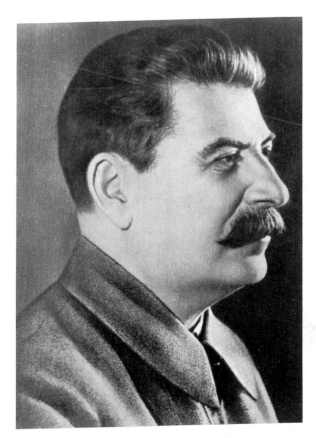

Fig. 10.1 Joseph Vissarionovich Stalin (1878–1953). After the death of Vladimir Lenin, Stalin moved quickly to establish and consolidate his power as dictator of the Soviet Union. In the 1930s, he instigated purges of the Communist Party, which led to the execution, imprisonment, and exile of many Soviet citizens. Concerning the exercise of power, Stalin is reputed once to have said, "The death of one man is a tragedy, but the death of millions a statistic"

people with a vision for their organization and a strong belief that they are the right people to lead its pursuit.

One of the greatest sources of power any leader enjoys is the ability to regulate the access to power of other members of the organization. For example, a chair may withhold or reallocate key information in ways that reduce the ability of certain colleagues to influence others in the department. Such information could include strategic plans, financial data, and impending personnel changes. By disseminating such information through an acknowledged management structure, a chain of command, or responsibility, that structure tends to be reinforced, while circumventing it tends to undermine it.

It is important to note that the lines of authority in every organization are both formal and informal. Colleagues with little formal, legitimate power may nonetheless exercise substantial informal, referent power through sheer force of personality, depth of vision, and personal loyalty. For example, former department chairs or deans may wield considerable influence, even though they no longer retain any formal authority.

Of course, merely possessing power is not enough to lead effectively. We must also know how to exercise power effectively in the pursuit of the goals of the organization and the profession. Like power itself, the effective exercise of power is context-dependent and varies from organization to organization, depending on a variety of personal, social, and political circumstances. Leading a group of people such as physicians, who highly esteem prerogatives such as autonomy and prestige, may call for different leadership approaches than leading the housekeeping department. Furthermore, what works in one department or institution may not work in another, and even the most perfectly adapted approach will not work indefinitely, as circumstances change. By developing a schema of the different types of organizational challenges leaders confront, it is possible to define more clearly the optimal strategies for meeting each one.

Hershey and colleagues developed a situational model of leadership that begins with three distinct leadership factors. These are task behavior, relationship behavior, and follower readiness. Task behavior refers to a leader's work in organizing personnel and responsibilities to achieve the organization's objectives, including ongoing guidance and direction in these matters. Relationship behavior concerns the leader's personal interactions with members of the organization, such as communicating openly with followers and supporting them in their personal and professional pursuits. Follower readiness refers to the propensity of colleagues to perform necessary tasks and to pursue the organization's objectives.

Of these three factors, the key one is follower readiness. The appropriate leadership approach in any organizational setting depends on the readiness of subordinates to follow the lead of the leader. There are four fundamental decision-making strategies the leader may adopt, and the one chosen depends primarily on the level of follower readiness. There are telling, selling, participatory decision making, and delegating.

The first strategy is telling colleagues what to do. In this scenario, the leader makes the decision alone, with no involvement of colleagues. The leader decides who should do what and directs them in doing so. This type of leadership involves a high degree of task behavior and a low degree of relationship behavior. Such an approach might make sense if colleagues are both unable and unwilling to pursue the needs of an educational program and the leader makes the determination that cultivating their support is either impractical or undesirable.

Generally speaking, telling will not be an effective strategy for leading physicians and medical educators. Crisis situations may warrant such an approach, because they may not allow much time for decision making, rendering it impossible to invite participation, build support, or even explain decisions. We should not convene a study group or a committee when the fire alarm sounds. However, making telling a habit suggests that the leader is an autocrat, and that the organization is being so poorly managed that it exists in a perpetual crisis mentality.

The strategy of selling decisions means the leader decides and attempts to solicit support. This style involves both high task behavior and high relationship behavior. Leaders still need to explain the task and how to accomplish it, but they wish to create enthusiasm among colleagues to get the job done as quickly and effectively as possible. In contrast to telling, selling involves a greater degree of interest in colleagues as persons, and is likely to prove offensive to colleagues who highly value autonomy. On the other hand, selling imposes a greater expenditure of time and effort in implementing decisions. Selling is likely to make sense in situations where leaders know what needs to be done but wish to develop support within the organization for doing it. Suppose the dean has told a department chair that a new method of evaluating medical students must be introduced in all the department's courses. It would be foolish and even misleading for the chair to pretend to involve colleagues in debate over whether to introduce the new evaluation system. However, the chair might get department members involved in determining its benefits and costs, and developing an implementation plan. This might, in turn, foster a more participatory frame of mind that enhances commitment to the new system.

In participatory decision making, leaders invite colleagues to take part in decision making and share responsibility with them for developing a course of action. This involves a relatively low level of task behavior on the part of the leader, but a high level of relationship behavior. Participatory decision making tends to work best in situations where leaders are either unsure which decision is best or believe that collaboration will produce a better decision than any single leader could produce. High relationship behavior is important because it encourages colleagues to come together and helps to secure their support both for the decision-making process and its final product.

The participatory approach is not suited to all situations. For example, suppose the stakes are very low, colleagues possess little or no expertise in the matter at hand or a participatory process is likely either to take too long or to prove too arduous.

When the leader simply allows colleagues to make the decision, the approach is delegating. It is characterized by both low-task and low-relationship behavior, as the leader stays out of the process and provides little guidance or encouragement. Delegation is possible in situations where colleagues are able and willing to take responsibility for decision making. In other words, follower readiness must be high. In such situations, following another approach would only slow the process and risk producing resentment among colleagues. Delegation also works well where the organization's stake in a decision is low and there is little potential for harm, regardless of what decision is reached. Leaders who impose themselves on every decision risk expending valuable leadership capital while simultaneously acquiring a reputation for meddlesomeness. A key trait of effective leaders is knowing when to get out of the way.

Developed by Robert House and Terence Mitchell, the path–goal theory of leadership provides further guidance on which leadership approaches are likely to be effective in different organizational contexts. Like the situational model just described, path–goal theory emphasizes the importance of the organizational context of leadership. It also holds that the situation at hand powerfully determines the extent of the leader's influence on events using different approaches. Using a medical analogy, the leader needs to identify correctly the organizational situation (diagnosis) before it is possible to choose the leadership approach (therapy) most appropriate to it.

The leader functions by helping to define a goal for the organization's members and a path by which that goal can be achieved. Anything that helps colleagues to understand better the objectives they are pursuing, pursue them with greater vigor, or increase their sense of reward with the result can powerfully contribute to the achievement of the organization's mission. The path–goal theory posits four fundamental types of leadership conduct, each of which is best suited to different situations: directive leadership, supportive leadership, participatory leadership, and achievement-oriented leadership.

Directive leadership builds on the leader's function of initiating structure. Directive leaders set the goal, provide instructions for pursuing it, and monitor progress. Directive leadership best suits organizations where members are poorly prepared for the task at hand or the nature of the work is highly routine or unstructured. Highly educated professionals such as physicians and medical educators are unlikely to respond well to directive leadership unless they are faced with ambiguous tasks with which they have little experience. The dean or department chair who directs colleagues in the details of arranging their daily schedules is likely to produce dissatisfaction and dissent.

Supportive leadership involves a primarily relationship approach focused on building mutually rewarding relationships and tending to the personal, social, and organizational well-being of others. Supportive leadership is most appropriate in situations where colleagues clearly understand the nature of their work. When the goal and task are clear, there is little need for directive leadership. The leader's primary function is to ensure that everyone gets along and remains motivated to accomplish the organization's objectives. An example would be the day-to-day work of teaching in a medical school. If everyone is doing well, tending to interpersonal relationships and building and maintaining morale are key to fostering continued excellence.

Participatory leadership involves actively consulting with colleagues, seeking their suggestions and advice, and involving them directly in the decision-making process. This approach works best in situations where the task and goals are somewhat ambiguous and followers have limited experience in carrying them out. For example, securing new leadership often works best when a search committee is formed, which makes it possible to capitalize on the personal and professional insights of colleagues regarding each candidate's strengths and weaknesses, as well as overall suitability for the position. Interaction between such committees and organizational leaders also often helps to clarify organizational objectives. To forgo a participatory approach in such situations cannot only compromise performance but undermine morale by denying colleagues a meaningful role in shaping the organization.

Achievement-oriented leadership means establishing challenging objectives and then expecting colleagues to perform up to their potential. Achievement-oriented approaches are best suited to situations of substantial organizational change, which place a premium on innovations that highly educated and experienced colleagues are often capable of providing. If a situation involves demands that are beyond the capabilities of colleagues, then achievement-oriented approaches are very likely to fail. This approach is also poorly suited to situations that pose little challenge. Challenging colleagues to accomplish things they already do every day would seem like a vote of no-confidence in their abilities and would rapidly prove counterproductive.

Educational Strategy

A transatlantic jet airliner entered a large storm system where it was buffeted about by strong winds. During the most intense turbulence, the passengers were startled to hear an explosion in the cockpit. Minutes later, the copilot's voice was heard over the intercom:

> Ladies and gentlemen, we have sustained damage to our equipment as a result of the storm. I have good news and bad news. The bad news is that our plane's navigational system is ruined and we do not know in what direction we are traveling. The good news is that we are experiencing strong tailwinds, and we are making record time.

Sadly, this story rings true for many educational leaders, who find themselves tossed about in a sea of turbulent change in medical education. Some of us have been working so hard just to keep our program's head above water that we have little energy left to think about where the currents are carrying us. Treading water is simply no way to navigate: you get nowhere, you soon grow exhausted, and you end up drowning anyway. As educational leaders, we cannot afford to neglect two crucial questions: where we want to go, and how we are going to get there.

The future of medical education hinges on the quality of our leaders' strategic planning. We need to cultivate a strategic outlook, a type of outlook not always found in the framework of medical science or clinical medicine. This means critically examining our own assumptions and biases. It means not only asking, "What is?" but also, "What if?" We need to develop and sustain an ongoing dynamic interchange between medicine and the broader world, expanding educators' and learners' notions of relevance to encompass information that is not only accurate but thought provoking.

The benefits of a strategic approach in medical education are manifold. It enables us to develop a well-grounded identity, and fosters consistency in decision making and the identification of clearly specified goals. It encourages us to study the present situation in light of our aspirations for the future, helping us to determine where innovation is most vital. It requires us to communicate, both among ourselves and with colleagues in other organizations. It makes our programs and institutions more coherent and cohesive wholes. Finally, it may improve financial performance, by fostering greater coordination between goals and resources. Often the strategic plan itself is less important than the process of sharing perspectives and developing new ideas.

What are the elements of a strategic plan? Moving from top to bottom, they include mission, vision, strategy, goals, and actions. The mission of an organization is its reason for being. One of the most damning criticisms we could level at any educational program is that it lacks a mission. Without a mission, an organization does not know what it is ultimately trying to do. It is like an airliner whose pilot keeps it airborne, but is not proceeding toward any particular destination.

Nearly as bad as lacking a mission entirely is failing to ensure that all the members of the organization know the mission. If we do not know how our jobs fit into the overall purpose of the organization, then our ability to contribute to its achievement is severely compromised. If we do not know the mission, see it clearly, and pursue it enthusiastically, then we are unlikely to excel in our work. We need to believe that the world would be a poorer place without our work. Vision is the organization's mental picture of what it is trying to become in the future. The mission provides a frame of reference for the vision, but mission alone is not enough, because it does not specify how the organization's purposes are going to be achieved. If the mission tells why we need to erect a new building, the vision describes what the building will actually look like, based on the purpose it is being built to serve. The vision gives members of the organization a sense of what they are supposed to be moving toward, and thereby creates a sense of progress. It is important periodically to check the vision against the mission, to ensure that the organization's future faithfully reflects its reason for being. For example, do we educate our medical students with the intention that they pass all the standardized tests, or are we attempting to train first-rate physicians?

Strategy is the plan for achieving the vision. It is not enough to know what our educational programs are attempting to become. We must also understand how they are going to do so. There are many possible routes by which to reach a particular destination, and strategy considers such factors as effectiveness and efficiency in choosing among them. Effectiveness is the probability that we will reach the destination. Efficiency is the amount of resources we expend in doing so. The fact that efficiency appears only at the level of strategy, subordinate to mission and vision, highlights the secondary nature of its role in strategic planning. We must first determine why the medical school exists, then we can determine what resources it needs to accomplish its mission. Efficiency calculations can help determine what route to take, but they cannot specify what should be the destination.

Goals are specific targets for achieving the organization's vision. If strategy is the route the organization chooses to reach its destination, then goals are like the steps that must be taken along the way to get there, such as specific legs of the journey and stops for rest and refueling. A common strategy for formulating goals is to step back from time to time and construct top five lists of key targets that must be reached if the organization is to realize its vision. Generally, such goals should be outlined at least annually, and more often in environments that invite rapid change. Of course, goals must not be written in stone, and should be subject to change as circumstances demand. In the absence of clearly defined goals, however, even the most visionary strategic plan will produce little in the way of results, because no one sees what to do now to move the organization along.

Actions are specific tasks that must be accomplished to achieve goals. For example, while driving along the leg of a particular journey, it is necessary to turn the steering wheel, sometimes to the right and other times to the left, in order to avoid crashing. In organizations, such tasks must be assigned to particular individuals, have clearly defined time frames, and specify both authority and accountability for their completion. By planning actions appropriately, it is possible to build short-term successes into longer-term strategic plans, thereby fostering morale and momentum throughout a lengthy strategic course.

Permeating all levels of the strategic plan are the organization's ethical principles. Ethical principles are our moral compass, our sense of what kind of an organization we are and what we will and will not do in pursuit of our objectives. Ethical principles powerfully affect the organization's performance because they define our basic way of doing business. How are our targets formulated, how do we reward ourselves, how do we handle disagreements, and so on? Do we allow faculty members to publicly berate medical students or residents? What are learners supposed to do if they encounter a situation that makes them ethically uncomfortable? Who are our role models, and what do they exemplify? Such principles set a tone throughout the organization, and making sure the best principles are in place is one of the most important missions of educational leaders.

The word strategy is drawn from a Greek root that refers to leading an army, and a synonym for strategy in this sense would be generalship. In military parlance, strategy is distinguished from tactics. Generally speaking, tactics refer to decision making that takes place once the enemy has been engaged, whereas strategy refers to planning that takes place prior to engagement. During the Second World War, the USA and its allies engaged in strategic bombing of German industries such as petroleum refining and manufacturing, in an effort to undermine the German capacity to wage war. Most battles are decided before the first shot is ever fired.

The resources of every organization are limited, and one mission of strategic planning is to plan the allocation of those limited resources in a way that produces the maximum medium-term and long-term payoffs. Many of us spend too much time thinking tactically, taxing our ingenuity to solve problems as they arise in daily work. By dint of years of experience in the trenches, we become quite good at bandaging wounds, but too often we fail to step back and examine the system that repeatedly gives rise to the injuries in the first place. The strategic approach is to step back and think creatively about how to improve the system, be it a particular process or the whole organization. It means asking radical questions about why the system is composed and structured as it is, and whether it really ought to remain that way.

Physicians tend to be a fairly conservative group. Since our first days in medical school, we were reminded again and again of the Hippocratic maxim, "First do no harm." Eager to excel, we became adept at recalling what our teachers told us to learn, a pattern that often continues and intensifies during residency training. Creativity is not a priority. Ask most medical students or residents what we want to learn, and we will point to a textbook. The implicit message? Learn everything, and do not get caught not knowing something. Our curriculum is more conducive to conformity than creativity, despite the fact that the latter is greatly needed.

The future of medical education does not depend on cultivating leaders who are so careful they never make mistakes. Quite the opposite; the future of medical education, and ultimately that of the whole profession of medicine, depends on cultivating leaders with the courage to take risks, the judgment to know which risks are worth taking, and the ability to learn from mistakes. Show me a department chair or a dean who never makes mistakes, and I will show you an organization in desperate need of new leadership. If we adopt a defensive posture and attempt to insulate ourselves from change, we become mere stepping-stones for innovators who are eager to blaze new trails.

Among the greatest enemies of innovation are complacency and fear. Good enough is the enemy of better, and academic physicians who are satisfied with the status quo are unlikely to attempt to enhance performance. Every one of us has colleagues whose attitude toward the future is one of trepidation. Their perspective may be likened to that of Lord Salisbury, who argued that whatever happens will be for the worse, so it is best that as little happen as possible. They regard strategic planning warily. As long as such individuals regard the unknown as more threatening than the status quo, meaningful innovation will be impossible.

Leaders need imagination, the ability to foresee a future better than the present, or at least better than the current trajectory. And one key attribute of imaginative leaders is openness. Getting people to do what we want is less important than the ability to listen to what others have to contribute and put it to good use. In the knowledge economy, freedom and creativity become increasingly important, and they require an open exchange of ideas and perspectives. The totalitarian state, as embodied in the former Soviet bloc, illustrates the antithesis of a model of effective leadership, in which conformity underwritten by the threat of force was prized above all. In the future of medical schools, outstanding leaders will be defined not by how much power they wield but by how much they know, and how much they know will depend on how well they listen.

To be successful, we need to promote and encourage conversation. Most leaders are overburdened with information, but starved for genuine perspective. In what new and fruitful ways could we think about our organization and its mission? We need to become the number one connoisseurs and disseminators of new perspectives. We need to build cultures where everyone at every level is encouraged to learn and to share what they know. Effective strategic planning requires inclusiveness, taking advantage of as many perspectives as possible. Especially helpful are colleagues who help us to see problems and opportunities in new ways. The last thing we need is yes-men. Such people merely confirm our prejudices. Instead, we need people who help us to reexamine our assumptions and biases.

An insulated leader is an ineffective leader. We need constant exposure to new ways of thinking, especially those from outside our field. The solutions to the most important problems rarely lie within the perspective of the people who first recognized them. We need to spend time reading and attending conferences outside our field. We might enroll in courses in other disciplines. The muscle of creativity is strengthened by such interdisciplinary experience. When it is not challenged, that muscle grows weak and flabby.

Creative leadership requires a questioning attitude. People who think they have everything figured out are the last ones to ask questions. Only through continuous inquiry can leaders ensure that organizational strategy is appropriately tuned to the true state of affairs. Every important decision involves uncertainty, but intelligent questioning can reduce that uncertainty to more manageable levels by providing a clearer conception of what the world really looks like.

Risk and reward are tightly correlated. As a consequence, we view uncertainty not as a handicap, leading to a paralysis of judgment, but as an opportunity for innovation, with substantial rewards for the organization. If there were no uncertainty, every program would thrive to the same extent as every other. Because uncertainty is always present, the best leaders are able to use superior understanding to full advantage. The organizations most likely to thrive are those whose vision extends beyond the box of conventional assumptions and who effectively integrate that vision into their strategic planning.

Socrates famously declared that the unexamined life is not worth living. Certainly the success of academic departments and medical schools that do not engage in frequent self-examination is likely to prove short lived. Such self-examination requires above all a willingness to acknowledge and redress deficiencies. The inability of academic physicians to face up to our mistakes sentences our programs to years of underachievement, our potential for flourishing largely untapped. Everything we do needs to be scrutinized, to determine whether current performance is in line with potential achievement. Mistakes are not signs that we should give up but laboratories of success. We need to cultivate a culture where mistakes are not only tolerated but welcomed. If we are not making mistakes from time to time, we are not learning, and if we are not learning from small mistakes, bigger and more catastrophic failures become inevitable.

Educating for Leadership

The late John Gardner, who served as US Secretary of Health, Education, and Welfare, argued that the professions do a poor job of developing leadership potential. In his book, *On Leadership*, Gardner declared that "the best learners are carefully schooled to avoid leadership responsibilities…. All over this country trouble is brewing, while our patterns of social and professional organization keep able and gifted potential leaders on the sidelines." The timeliness of Gardner's diagnosis is reflected in a spate of recent articles decrying the epidemic of apathy in medicine, particularly physicians' declining interest in serving in leadership capacities in private and academic practices and professional organizations. Why are not more future physicians committed to developing their own leadership capabilities to better serve their patients, communities, and profession?

One explanation for the dearth of interest and commitment to leadership among future physicians would be that they are either lazy or simply do not care sufficiently for their organizations and the field to make a commitment to leadership. Another explanation, the one I prefer, is Gardner's; namely, the fact that we often fail to do a good job of preparing future physicians to lead. After all, most medical students and residents spend thousands of hours learning to collect information, offer differential diagnoses, and make recommendations for diagnostic testing and therapy. By contrast, leadership is not a topic in many medical school and residency curricula, and knowledge and skills in this area are generally not prerequisites for professional credentialing or advancement.

What would happen if we made leadership a formal part of the curriculum, or at least an option for interested learners? Could we develop a curriculum of basic leadership knowledge and skills? Could we get commitments to free learners from other clinical and training responsibilities on a regular basis to participate in such a program? Would we be able to identify a group of learners with sufficient interest in leadership development to volunteer to take part in such a program, and faculty to lead it? And even if the answers to all these questions were in the affirmative, would the learners who participated in such a program judge that it had truly enhanced their interest and aptitude for leadership?

Particularly at times of rapid change in healthcare, the need for top-notch physician leadership in group practices, hospitals, healthcare organizations, and health policy debates is great. Yet over the long term, physicians have been playing a shrinking leadership role. For example, over the past 75 years, the percentage of US hospitals that have a physician chief executive has diminished from 35% to fewer than 4%. Hospitals have moved away from, rather than toward, leadership by patient-care professionals. The reasons for this shift are complex, but one of the most important is the fact that, in contrast to business schools, medical schools and residency programs often ignore leadership and do a poor job of developing leadership potential.

Medicine is under intense scrutiny by healthcare organizations and policymakers, who frequently have little appreciation for what physicians do. We are fortunate that medicine attracts some of the brightest and best college students year after year, but it is vital that more medical schools and residency programs recognize the need for leadership and take steps to develop some of these highly capable people as future leaders. The first step in doing so is to put leadership on the map, by promoting it as an important ability, providing meaningful training and experience in this area, and recognizing and rewarding residents who take up the challenge.

An intense focus on leadership is not for everyone, and it would be both undesirable and impossible for every future physician to become a section chief, department chair, group president, hospital CEO, or dean. Yet every physician functions as a leader in numerous ways, not least with patients and families. Even physicians who never hold a formal office in an organization still lead in their facilities and communities. We are constantly shaping others' expectations, meeting or failing to meet those expectations, and generally speaking, creating the future of our field. In terms of formal leadership, the future of our departments, professional organizations, and the field itself hinges, in large part, on the quality of leadership they enjoy.

To foster leadership development, I advocate a two-tiered approach. First, all learners should be exposed to some lectures and discussions around leadership, perhaps just a few per year. Topics could include challenges and opportunities facing medicine or particular medical fields today, the perspectives and techniques of effective leaders, local and national leadership development and service opportunities, and opportunities to discuss the importance of leadership with people working on the front lines. This would help to ensure that leadership is on every learner's radar screen. Moreover, it would also serve as an entrée into additional leadership development opportunities for that subset of learners who are sufficiently intrigued to want to pursue it further.

Those learners who identify leadership as a special interest could then be offered the opportunity to participate in a more focused leadership development program. I am not suggesting that residents who choose leadership should devote a large percentage of their time, at the expense of clinical training, nor that they should forsake plans to pursue further education in a particular field of medicine to focus on leadership.

As an example, learners might meet once or twice per month. They could complete assigned readings on leadership, meet with experienced leaders from both inside and outside their organization to discuss leadership, and undertake practical leadership projects. Readings might consist of articles and books in medicine, healthcare, and leadership studies, including both case studies and more general topics such as motivation, communication, strategic planning, negotiation, assessment, and dealing with difficult people. Participants could complete the readings prior to meetings and come prepared to pose questions about the topic and identify applications of the material in their daily work lives.

Discussions with leaders could consist of three principal components. First, leaders could describe their own education and career with a view to illuminating their own path into leadership. This would help participants to understand how leadership opportunities arise. Second, leaders could discuss some of the leadership challenges they have faced recently and how they dealt with them. Ideally, some leaders would be willing to discuss not only their triumphs but also their failures and what they learned from them. Finally, learners could have an opportunity to pose questions to the leaders on whatever subjects they choose. In addition, leaders might offer a presentation or two for the entire learning community, helping to highlight leadership even for learners and educators who are not formal participants in the leadership program.

Learners could also develop their own projects, to be pursued with the assistance of a faculty mentor. In some cases, participants might choose to work on a solo project, while in others they might elect to work in pairs or groups. The goal of the projects would be to enable learners to gain practical experience in investigating and formulating a response to a real-world challenge facing their organization. Examples of topics that might be addressed include some aspect of the educational program, a scheduling system, a means of assessing productivity or performance, and an approach to improving clinical workflow or decreasing error rates. One of the keys to success of such projects is that they should be both clearly defined and eminently feasible. The goal is not to solve all the world's problems, but to make real headway in addressing one of them.

Of course, presentations, articles, and books on leadership do not necessarily translate into improvements in the quality of leadership. Most medical learners are strongly focused on developing their clinical acumen. They may regard the demands of clinical training as so great that they do not seek out learning opportunities in such areas. For leadership to come to life and begin to shape the way we educate future physicians, we need to make it a formal part of medical education. If we want leadership to be part of learners' aspirations, we need to include it on our educational programs.